# Localization of Putative Steroid Receptors

## Volume II
## Clinically Oriented Studies

Editors

**Louis P. Pertschuk, D.O.**
Associate Professor
Department of Pathology
State University of New York
Downstate Medical Center
and
Attending Pathologist
Department of Pathology
Kings County Hospital Center
Brooklyn, New York

**Sin Hang Lee, M.D., F.R.C.P.(C)**
Attending Pathologist
Department of Pathology
Hospital of St. Raphael
and
Associate Clinical Professor
Department of Pathology
Yale University School of Medicine
New Haven, Connecticut

CRC Press, Inc.
Boca Raton, Florida

**Library of Congress Cataloging in Publication Data**
Main entry under title:

Localization of putative steroid receptors.

  Bibliography: p.
  Includes index.
  Contents: v. 1. Experimental systems — v. 2.
Clinically oriented studies.
  1. Cancer—Endocrine aspects. 2. Steroid hormones—
Receptors. I. Pertschuk, Louis P., 1925-
II. Lee, Sin Hang, 1932- . [DNLM: 1. Receptors,
Steroid—analysis. 2. Histocytochemistry—methods.
3. Breast Neoplasms—analysis. WK 150 L811]
RC268.2.L63   1985   616.99'449071   84-20049
ISBN 0-8493-6048-X (v. 1)
ISBN 0-8493-6049-8 (v. 2)

Direct all inquiries to CRC Press, Inc., 2000 Corporate Blvd., N.W., Boca Raton, Florida, 33431.

© 1985 by CRC Press, Inc.

International Standard Book Number 0-8493-6048-X  (Volume I)
International Standard Book Number 0-8493-6049-8  (Volume II)

Library of Congress Card Number 84-20049
Printed in the United States

# PREFACE

For the past two decades, the study of steroid hormone receptors has been almost entirely pursued by investigators whose primary expertise has been in the field of steroid biochemistry. To these workers, who have contributed so much of the information upon which our present knowledge is based, the medical and scientific communities are greatly indebted.

However, for a full understanding of the mechanism of steroid action at the cellular level, it has become necessary to know not only the precise cells in which steroids exert their effects, but also the subcellular compartments in which the specific steroid binding proteins are concentrated. Since biochemical assays are performed on homogenized tissue extracts, they possess certain inherent limitations. In addition, as sophisticated equipment is required for their performance, there are large areas of the world in which they cannot be performed. Therefore many patients (in particular with breast cancer) are unable to reap the benefits which might accrue if information about tumor receptors was available.

The past few years have witnessed the development of morphologic assays designed to assess steroid hormone binding. The prime purpose of these techniques (since they are performed on intact tissue sections) has been to obtain information not readily gleaned from conventional assays. Of more importance, most are designed in such a manner that they could be executed in any hospital pathology laboratory. Many of the morphologic assays covered in this work have been developed by pathologists, often with considerable service duties related to patient care, and in many cases without research funds. It is not surprising that these assays have become subjects of much criticism. Nonetheless, as evidenced throughout this work, a number of enthusiastic researchers have obtained quite impressive results and countered much of the criticism. More recently, some research laboratories specializing in steroid biochemistry have also begun to direct an increasing share of effort and resources towards the development of morphological assays, including the use of monoclonal antibodies which can trace receptor antigens *in situ*. As a consequence, there no longer exists a sharp boundary between the fields of biochemistry and pathology.

These volumes represent the "state-of-the-art" in morphological methods for detection of steroid receptors. No final solution is presented or intended. Indeed, at present a definite answer to the question "where is the receptor located?" cannot be given. Furthermore, there are a number of discrepancies, some serious, which prevail.

In Volume I we have attempted to collect current available methods and experimental approaches which might be useful in solving present enigmas. Some physician authors, not being content to wait until complete answers are available, have applied many of the new methodologies in clinical research projects designed to improve medical practice. These attempts we have placed in Volume II. Of necessity, there is occasional overlap with newer techniques and experimental data in the latter volume.

It is our hope that the background and recent advances presented here will stimulate further experimentation and new innovations, and spur clinical trials by all investigators with an interest in steroid hormones, cell biology, and clinical oncology.

**Louis P. Pertschuk**
**Sin Hang Lee**

# THE EDITORS

**Louis P. Pertschuk, D. O.,** is Associate Professor of Pathology at State University of New York, Downstate Medical Center, and Attending Pathologist at the Kings County Hospital Center, Brooklyn, New York.

Dr. Pertschuk received an A.B. in Biology from New York University in 1946 and graduated from the Philadelphia College of Osteopathic Medicine in 1950. Following a year of internship he entered private general practice until 1970 when he began a residency in pathology at the State University-Kings County Hospital Center. He was a Fellow in Pathology at the Memorial Sloan-Kettering Cancer Center in 1973 and 1974 and was certified in Anatomic Pathology by the American Board of Pathology in 1974.

Dr. Pertschuk is a Fellow of the College of American Pathologists and the American Society of Clinical Pathology. He is a member of the American Association of Pathologists, the International Academy of Pathology, the New York Academy of Sciences, and the American Association for the Advancement of Science. He has published 67 research papers, 43 scientific abstracts, and contributed 19 chapters to various books. His current research interests include the development and study of different methodologies for detection of the sites of action of steroid hormones, especially in human neoplasia.

**Sin Hang Lee, M.D.,** is Attending Pathologist at the Hospital of St. Raphael, and an Associate Clinical Professor of Pathology at Yale University in New Haven, Connecticut.

Born in Hong Kong, Dr. Lee is a 1956 graduate of Wuhan Medical College, the People's Republic of China. After graduation, he worked in Sichuan Medical College, China, as a microbiologist before he joined the Department of Pathology at the University of Hong Kong in 1961 as a demonstrator. He finished his residency in pathology in the U.S. at the New York Hospital-Cornell Medical Center, and was appointed Instructor in Pathology at Cornell Medical College in 1966. In the same year, he was certified by the American Board of Pathology, and was made a Fellow of the Royal College of Physicians of Canada. Dr. Lee spent the year of 1967 to 1968 as a Pathology Fellow at Memorial Hospital for Cancer and Allied Diseases. Thereafter, he served as Assistant Professor of Pathology at McGill University (1968 to 1971) and subsequently Associate Professor of Pathology at Yale University (1971 to 1973). In addition to the current hospital and academic appointments in New Haven, Dr. Lee also holds a guest professorship at Wuhan Medical College, the People's Republic of China.

Dr. Lee's professional and research interests range from surgical pathology to electron microscopic localization of enzymes and mycoplasma antigens. As a surgical pathologist, he saw an urgent need for a practical histochemical approach to the identification of breast cancer cells rich in estrogen receptors, and has devoted much of his free time during the past few years to develop the hydrophilic fluorescent estradiol technique, which has become the most popular histochemical assay of estrogen receptors to date.

# CONTRIBUTORS

**J.P.A. Baak, M.D., Ph.D.**
Pathological Institute
Free University Hospital
Amsterdam, The Netherlands

**Alberto Bagni, M.D.**
Resident in Pathology
Department of Pathological Anatomy and
 Histopathology
University of Ferrara
Ferrara, Italy

**Etienne-Emile Baulieu, M.D., Ph.D.**
Professor
Department of Biochemistry
University of Paris South
Bicetre, France

**Christopher C. Benz, M.D.**
Assistant Professor of Medicine
Cancer Research Institute
University of California at San Francisco
San Francisco, California

**Maximilian Binder, Ph.D.**
Assistant Professor
Institute for Tumorbiology and Cancer
 Research
University of Vienna
Vienna, Austria

**Manfred Boehm, M.D.**
Research Associate
Institute for Tumorbiology and Cancer
 Research
University of Vienna
Vienna, Austria

**Richard H. Buell, M.D.**
Lady Davis Institue for Medical Research
Sir Mortimer B. Davis-Jewish General
 Hospital
Montreal, Quebec, Canada

**Giovanni Bussolati, M.D.**
Professor
Department of Pathology
University of Turin Medical School
Turin, Italy

**Anne C. Carter, M.D.**
Visiting Professor
Department of Medicine
Division of Endocrinology
State University of New York
Downstate Medical Center
Brooklyn, New York

**Peizhen Chen, M.D.**
Associate Professor
Department of Surgery
Sichuan Medical College
Chengdu, Sichuan, China

**Klaus Czerwenka, M.D.**
Head, Department of Gynecology and
 Obstetrics
Histology and Cytology Unit
University of Vienna
Vienna, Austria

**Karen S. Byer Eisenberg, R.N.,
M.P.S.**
Assistant Nursing Director
Department of Pathology
State University of New York
Downstate Medical Center
Brooklyn, New York

**Vincenzo Eusebi, M.D.**
Associate Professor
Department of Pathology
University of Bologna Medical School
Bologna, Italy

**Guidalberto Fabris, M.D.**
Associate Professor
Department of Pathological Anatomy and
 Histopathology
University of Ferrara
Ferrara, Italy

**Joseph G. Feldman, M.D.**
Associate Professor
Department of Preventive Medicine
State University of New York
Downstate Medical Center
Brooklyn, New York

**Bernard Fisher, M.D.**
Professor of Surgery
Department of Surgery
University of Pittsburgh School of
  Medicine
Pittsburgh, Pennsylvania

**Jean-Marie Gasc, Ph.D.**
Maitre-Assistant
Institute of Embryology
Nogent-sur-Marne, France

**N. Gunduz, Ph.D.**
Assistant Professor of Surgical Research
Department of Surgery
University of Pittsburgh School of
  Medicine
Pittsburgh, Pennsylvania

**Wedad Hanna, M.D., F.R.C.P.(C)**
Assistant Professor
Department of Pathology
University of Toronto
Staff Pathologist
Women's College Hospital
Toronto, Ontario, Canada

**David L. Ingram, A.A.P.A.**
Research Assistant, Pathology Associate
Department of Pathology
Duke University Medical Center
Durham, North Carolina

**Raimund Jakesz, M.D.**
Assistant Professor
Department of Surgery
University of Vienna
Vienna, Austria

**Charmayne Jesik, Ph.D.**
Research Associate
Department of Urology
Northwestern University Medical School
Chicago, Illinois

**Roland Kolb, M.D.**
Associate Professor
Department of Surgery
University of Vienna
Vienna, Austria

**Pietro Lampertico, M.D.**
Head, Anatomical Pathology Laboratory
Unità Socio-Sanitaria Locale
Busto Arsizio, Italy

**Chung Lee, Ph.D.**
Associate Professor
Department of Urology
Northwestern University Medical School
Chicago, Illinois

**J. Lindeman, M.D., Ph.D.**
Head, Department of Pathology
S.S.D.Z.
Delft, The Netherlands

**Richard J. Macchia, M.D.**
Associate Professor of Urology
Department of Urology
State University of New York
Downstate Medical Center
Brooklyn, New York

**Marayart Mangkornkanok**
Assistant Professor
Department of Pathology
Northwestern University Medical School
Chicago, Illinois

**Elisabetta Marchetti, M.D.**
Assistant Professor
Department of Pathological Anatomy and
  Histopathology
University of Ferrara
Ferrara, Italy

**Andrea Marzola, M.D.**
Associate Professor
Department of Pathological Anatomy and
  Histopathology
University of Ferrara
Ferrara, Italy

**Mauricio Maturana**
Mathematician and Statician
Institute of Public Health
University of Chile Medical School
Santiago, Chile

**Kenneth McCarty, Jr., M.D., Ph.D.**
Associate Professor of Pathology
Assistant Professor of Medicine
Duke University Medical Center
Durham, North Carolina

**Kenneth McCarty, Sr., Ph.D.**
Professor of Biochemistry
Duke University Medical Center
Durham, North Carolina

**Zhijia Mei, M.D.**
Instructor
Department of Oncology
Sichuan Medical College
Chengdu, Sichuan, China

**C.J.L.M. Meijer, M.D., Ph.D.**
Professor
Pathological Institute
Free University Hospital
Amsterdam, The Netherlands

**Miguel A. Mena**
Biologist
Laboratory of Experimental
  Endocrinology
Department of Experimental Morphology
University of Chile Medical School
Santiago, Chile

**Xiangin Meng, M.D.**
Associate Professor
Department of Pathology
Sichuan Medical College
Chengdu, Sichuan, China

**Italo Nenci, M.D.**
Professor of Pathology
Director, Department of Pathological
  Anatomy and Histopathology
University of Ferrara
Ferrara, Italy

**Kathleen I. Pritchard, M.D.,
  F.R.C.P.(C)**
Assistant Professor, Department of
  Medicine
University of Toronto
Staff Physician, Women's College
  Hospital
Toronto, Ontario, Canada

**Patrizia Querzoli, M.D.**
Resident in Pathology
Department of Pathological Anatomy and
  Histopathology
University of Ferrara
Ferrara, Italy

**Georg Reiner, M.D.**
Department of Surgery
University of Vienna
Vienna, Austria

**Angel Rodriguez**
Biologist
Laboratory of Experimental
  Endocrinology
Department of Experimental Morphology
University of Chile Medical School
Santiago, Chile

**Elizabeth A. Saffer, B.A.**
Senior Research Assistant
Department of Surgery
University of Pittsburgh School of
  Medicine
Pittsburgh, Pennsylvania

**Julia Sensibar, B.Sc.**
Research Assistant
Department of Urology
Northwestern University Medical School
Chicago, Illinois

**Juergen Spona, Ph.D.**
Head, Endocrine Research Unit
Department of Gynecology and Obstetrics
University of Vienna
Vienna, Austria

**Franca Stagni, D.Sc.**
Biologist
Anatomical Pathology Laboratory
Unità Socio-Sanitaria Locale
Busto Arsizio, Italy

**Andrei N. Tchernitchin, M.D.**
Head, Laboratory of Experimental
  Endocrinology
Department of Experimental Morphology
University of Chile Medical School
Santiago, Chile

**Gilles Tremblay, M.D.**
Senior Pathologist
Royal Victoria Hospital
Professor of Pathology
McGill University
Montreal, Quebec, Canada

**J. van Marle, Ph.D.**
Senior Scientist
Department of Pharmacology
University of Amsterdam
Amsterdam, The Netherlands

**Rosemary A. Walker, M.D.,
 M.R.C. Pathology**
Senior Lecturer
Department of Pathology
University of Leicester
Leicester, England

**Israel Wiznitzer, M.D.**
Postdoctoral Research Associate
Yale University School of Medicine
New Haven, Connecticut

**Xianyun Yao, M.D.**
Associate Professor
Department of Pathology
Sichuan Medical College
Chengdu, Sichuan, China

# TABLE OF CONTENTS

## Volume I: Experimental Systems

Chapter 1
An Overview ................................................................. 1
**S. H. Lee and L. P. Pertschuk**

Chapter 2
Radioautographic Localization of Estrogen Receptors in the Rat Uterus: a Tool for the Study
of Classical and Nontraditional Mechanisms of Hormone Action ........................ 5
**A. N. Tchernitchin, M. A. Mena, A. Rodriguez, and M. Maturana**

Chapter 3
Fluoresceinated Estrone Binding by Normal and Neoplastic Cells of Human and Animal
Origin ..................................................................... 39
**N. Gunduz, E. Saffer, and B. Fisher**

Chapter 4
Histochemical Study of Estrogen Receptors in the Rat Uterus With a Hydrophilic Fluorescent
Estradiol Conjugate ......................................................... 59
**S. H. Lee**

Chapter 5
Estrogen Receptors and Hormone Responsiveness in Serially Transplanted Mammary Tumors
in Rats ................................................................... 85
**C. Lee, C. Jesik, M. Mangkornkanok, J. Sensibar, and S. H. Lee**

Chapter 6
Flow Cytometric Analysis of Fluorescent Estrogen Binding in Cancer Cell
Suspensions ............................................................... 95
**C. Benz, I. Wiznitzer, and S. H. Lee**

Chapter 7
Sex Steroid Action Mechanism by Cytochemistry in Normal and Neoplastic
Target Tissues ............................................................ 111
**E. Marchetti, A. Marzola, A. Bagni, P. Querzoli, G. Fabris, and I. Nenci**

Chapter 8
Immunohistochemical Studies with Antibodies to the Chicken Oviduct
Progesterone Receptor ...................................................... 125
**J.-M. Gasc and E.-E. Baulieu**

Chapter 9
Methods for the Quantification of Histochemical Steroid Binding Assays .............. 143
**L. P. Pertschuk**

Chapter 10
A Two-State Immunocytochemical Method for Putative Estrogen Receptor Analysis .. 161
**V. Eusebi and G. Bussolati**

Chapter 11
Estradiol-BSA Conjugates for Estrogen Receptor Localization: the Vienna
Experience ............................................................... 167
**M. Binder, K. Czerwenka, M. Boehm, J. Spona, R. Jakesz, R. Kolb, and G. Reiner**

Index .................................................................... 183

# TABLE OF CONTENTS

## Volume II: Clinically Oriented Studies

Chapter 1
The Application of Thaw-Mount Autoradiography for the Localization of Putative Estrogen
Target Cells in Human Mammary Lesions ............................................. 1
**R. H. Buell and G. Tremblay**

Chapter 2
Morphologic Detection of Multiple Steroid Binding Sites in Breast Cancer by
Histochemistry and by Immunocytochemistry with Monoclonal Antireceptor Antibody:
Relationship to Endocrine Response.................................................... 15
**L. P. Pertschuk, K. B. Eisenberg, A. C. Carter, and J. G. Feldman**

Chapter 3
A Fluorescent Histochemical Study of Steroid Receptors in Human Breast Cancer...... 37
**S. H. Lee**

Chapter 4
Histochemical Sex Steroid Hormone Receptor Assay and Treatment of Breast Cancer
in Chinese Patients ..................................................................... 51
**P. Chen, X. Yao, Z. Mei, and X. Meng**

Chapter 5
Cancer of the Breast: Clinicopathological Correlations in Primary,, Recurrent, and Metastatic
Tumors with Histochemically Determined Hormone Receptors......................... 63
**P. Lampertico and F. Stagni**

Chapter 6
How to Validate Histochemical Techniques as Predictors of Hormonal Response ....... 85
**W. Hanna and K. I. Pritchard**

Chapter 7
Localization of Steroid Binding in Prostatic Carcinoma by Histochemistry:
Therapeutic Implications .............................................................. 93
**L. P. Pertschuk, R. J. Macchia, and K. B. Eisenberg**

Chapter 8
Binding of Labeled Estrogen-Albumin Conjugates in Breast Cancer ................... 113
**J. van Marle, J.P.A. Baak, C.J.L.M. Meijer, and J. Lindeman**

Chapter 9
Peroxidase Labeling of Estrogen Binding Sites in Breast Cancer...................... 133
**R. A. Walker**

Chapter 10
Critical Issues in the Evaluation of Histochemical and Biochemical Methods for
Steroid Receptor Analysis ............................................................ 149
**K. S. McCarty, Jr., D. L. Ingram, and K. S. McCarty, Sr.**

Index ................................................................................. 165

Chapter 1

# THE APPLICATION OF THAW-MOUNT AUTORADIOGRAPHY FOR THE LOCALIZATION OF PUTATIVE ESTROGEN TARGET CELLS IN HUMAN MAMMARY LESIONS*

**Richard H. Buell and Gilles Tremblay**

## TABLE OF CONTENTS

I.      Introduction................................................................. 2

II.     Materials and Methods....................................................... 2

III.    Results and Discussion...................................................... 3
        A.      Normal Mouse Tissues .............................................. 3
        B.      Human Tissue ..................................................... 5
                1.      Benign Lesions ........................................... 5
                2.      Malignant Lesions ........................................ 6

IV.     Conclusion................................................................. 10

References..................................................................... 11

*   Supported by a grant from the National Cancer Institute of Canada. During the course of this research RHB was supported by a fellowship from the Cancer Research Society of Montreal, Inc.

# I. INTRODUCTION

Interest has been stimulated among research groups to develop valid morphologic methods for localizing steroid hormone receptors in human breast cancer, because it is established that biochemical assays of these lesions are of proven prognostic value.[1] The major emphasis of research in this field has been directed towards methods with potential clinical application. Thus, many groups are investigating histochemical and immunocytochemical approaches, while there has been relatively little research on human tissue with autoradiographic methods, although these techniques were the first to be extensively investigated in experimental animals.

Autoradiographic techniques for localizing steroid hormone receptors were described in 1966 by Stumpf and Roth,[2] who showed that dry- and thaw-mount autoradiography yielded data that agreed well with biochemical assays. Indeed, it was Stumpf who in early work on the biochemical characterization of estrogen receptors (ER) provided autoradiographic evidence on the intracellular localization of these receptors.[3] Although the interpretation of some of this data has recently been questioned,[4,5] the methodology remains established as a means for localizing steroid binding sites in cells without artifactual diffusion of the ligand such as might occur with other methods employing fixation and dehydration of the specimens. Stumpf and co-workers have employed the methods successfully in a large series of studies on the localization of steroid target cells in experimental animals (for reviews see References 6 and 7). The methods are, however, relatively less practical in a clinical setting as in vitro incubation is necessary for the investigation of human tissue and only fresh biopsy specimens can be used. Nevertheless, autoradiographic methods have the distinct advantage of employing radioactive steroid ligands of known affinity for their receptors, and under appropriate conditions the results can be quantitated.[8-10] Because these ligands are used in biochemical investigations, much fundamental research relevant to the morphologic techniques has already been done and direct comparisons are feasible. Indeed, as Cunha et al. pointed out, with appropriate autoradiographic methods it may be possible to fulfill satisfactorily all generally accepted criteria for steroid-receptor binding, including quantifiable "saturation" analysis and high-affinity binding, and to correlate these morphologic observations with biochemical data.[9,10]

We have used thaw-mount autoradiography to investigate the distribution of putative estrogen target cells in human breast lesions, and, in this chapter, our findings will be summarized. The study initially involved experiments using the normal mouse uterus to establish the method.[11] Subsequently, we examined a series of human mammary lesions, both benign[12] and malignant.[13,14] Our results will be discussed in terms of the accuracy of the method and the possible biologic implications of our findings.

# II. MATERIALS AND METHODS

**Chemicals** — $[2,4,6,7]^3$H-estradiol (SA 90 or 102 Ci/mmol) was purchased from New England Nuclear Canada, Lachine, Quebec. It was purified by thin layer chromatography. Medium 199 with or without Hepes buffer was purchased from Grand Island Biological Co., Grand Island, N.Y. Nonradioactive steroids and other miscellaneous chemicals and reagents were purchased from Sigma Chemical Co., St. Louis, Mo. Kodak® NTB 2 emulsion and developing reagents were from Eastman Kodak, Montreal, Quebec. OCT compound for embedding tissues came from Lab Tek Products, Napierville, Ill. and liquid Freon 12 for freezing tissues was from Dupont, Canada.

**Tissues** — For in vivo studies and in vitro incubations of mouse uterus, 7- to 8-week female Balb/c mice were used. These were obtained either from a breeding colony maintained by Dr. G. Shyamala of the Lady Davis Institute of the Sir Mortimer B. Davis-Jewish General Hospital, Montreal or from the Canadian Breeding Farm, St. Constant, Quebec. The animals were kept under routine conditions. Each mouse was killed by cervical dislocation and the uterus or mammary tissue was removed within 5 to 10 min. Fresh human tissue, obtained at the time of frozen section examination, was transported to the laboratory in Medium 199 on ice. It was diced into pieces 1 to 2 mm thick.

**In vivo injections** — For in vivo injections mice were injected with 0.1 μg/20 g body weight $^3$H-estradiol. The animals were killed 2 hr after injection to allow sufficient time for radioactive steroid present in the blood to be cleared from the tissues.[15] After removal the tissue was diced into pieces 1 to 2 mm thick, embedded in OCT compound, and frozen immediately with liquid Freon 12. It was stored at $-76°C$ until sectioning, which was usually done within 2 weeks.

**In vitro incubation** — The method used for in vitro incubation of mouse uterus has been previously described[11] and will not be presented in detail. For human tissue,[12-14] 1-to 2-mm pieces were incubated at 30°C in Medium 199, pH 7.3, with a 5-n$M$ concentration of $^3$H-estradiol with or without a 100-fold excess of unlabeled estradiol or diethylstilbestrol (DES). The tissues were briefly blotted on filter paper, transferred to Medium 199 with 3.5 g % bovine serum albumin, and incubated for 2 to 4 hr. For benign tissues the incubation period was generally 3 hr, while for malignancies it was 4 hr. In all instances the mouse or human tissue was blotted again on filter paper after the incubation, embedded in OCT compound, frozen in liquid Freon 12, and stored at $-76°C$. Tissue sections were generally cut within 2 weeks of freezing.

**Thaw-mount autoradiography** — The thaw-mount autoradiographic procedure used is similar to the method originally described by Stumpf and Roth.[2] In a darkroom frozen sections of the tissue were cut at 4 μm and mounted onto glass slides previously coated with Kodak® NTB 2 emulsion. The sections were stored at $-15°C$ for the appropriate exposure time and then developed. Mouse tissues were stained with methyl green pyronin; human tissues were stained with hematoxylin and eosin.

**Identification of target cells** — The quantitative methods used for evaluation of data in the in vitro experiments with mouse uterus have been described and will not be discussed here.[11] For human tissues,[13] apparent target cells were identified by the predominance of nuclear grains in tissues exposed only to $^3$H-estradiol and the ability of radioinert estradiol or DES to suppress this labeling. For quantifying this subjective evaluation, a target cell was defined as one that demonstrated more than three times the average number of grains per 10 μm$^2$ nuclear cross-sectional area for 50 cells examined in tissue incubated with excess unlabeled inhibitor. For breast cancers,[14] a case was considered estrogen receptor-positive if: (1) the mean number of grains per 10 μm$^2$ nuclear cross-sectional area for 50 cells was greater for tissue exposed only to $^3$H-estradiol than for tissue also exposed to excess unlabeled estradiol or DES, and (2) at least 25% of the cells were considered target cells.

**Biochemical assay of breast cancers** — Biochemical assay of breast cancer tissue was done in the clinical laboratories of the Royal Victoria Hospital by established biochemical methods.[16] A case was positive if it contained more than 12 fmol/mg protein, borderline if it contained 6 to 12 fmol/mg protein, and negative if it contained less than 6 fmol/mg protein.

## III. RESULTS AND DISCUSSION

### A. Normal Mouse Tissues

In initial studies in vivo injections were done to determine the distribution of putative estrogen target cells in the mouse uterus and, in one instance, in the lactating mammary gland. The data from these experiments agreed with the observations of Sar and Stumpf.[7,17] The distribution of $^3$H-estradiol incorporation observed in the uterus was essentially the same

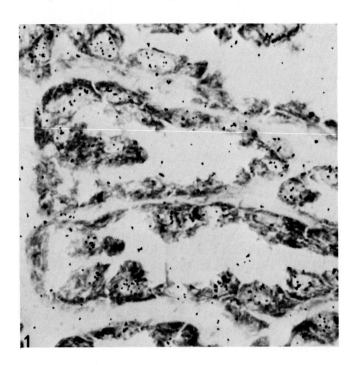

FIGURE 1.    Autoradiograph of mouse lactating mammary gland after in vivo injection of [3]H-estradiol. The figure demonstrates the nuclear retention of radioactivity in some but not all alveolar cells. (Methyl green pyronin; magnification × 680; 5 months exposure.)

as that seen after in vitro incubation and will be described below. In the lactating breast (Figure 1) uptake was identified in some but not all alveolar cells.

In the mouse uterus after in vitro incubation[11] (Figure 2), specific labeling, inhibited by radioinert estradiol or DES but not by progesterone or hydrocortisone, was identified in surface and glandular epithelium, stromal cells, and in the myometrial layer. Quantitation of the data revealed that differences in uptake observed between tissue incubated only in [3]H-estradiol and tissue incubated with excess unlabeled estradiol or DES were significant, but that progesterone had little effect in suppressing the observed labeling. In control experiments incubation of tissue in medium only and incubation of diaphragm in [3]H-estradiol revealed essentially no labeling at all.

In some cases the degree of labeling differed from area to area throughout the slide.[11] This observation is believed to represent an artifact of diffusion of the ligand or a relative difference in the efficiency of the albumin chase. The variation could be appreciated within a low-power field, but on high-power magnification the degree of labeling within given glands was similar, and in all cases specific labeling could be readily identified.

These studies were undertaken to assess the accuracy of an in vitro autoradiographic method for localizing putative estrogen target cells. It was evident from the results presented above that the binding sites identified were specific for estrogen and this labeling was absent in nontarget tissues. The binding was predominantly nuclear, as would be expected under these experimental conditions.[3-5,18] Whether with this technique the radioactive ligand can exchange with any endogenously bound radioinert estradiol was not determined, but Shannon et al.,[19] using a comparable in vitro incubation method with 17 n*M* [3]H-estradiol, did demonstrate such an exchange. The contribution to labeling from nuclear type II binding sites[20-22] was not investigated. If a portion of the observed label represented binding to these

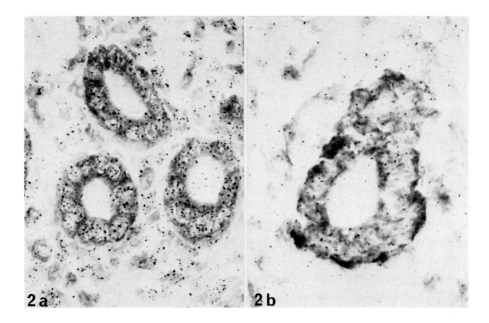

FIGURE 2.   (a) Autoradiograph of mouse uterus after in vitro incubation in [3]H-estradiol only. There is uptake and retention of [3]H-estradiol with predominant nuclear localization seen in most endometrial glandular cells and stromal cells. (Methyl green pyronin; magnification × 640; 34 days exposure.) (b) Portion of mouse uterus adjacent to that shown in Figure 2a. The section has been incubated in [3]H-estradiol with excess radioinert estradiol. The label seen is sparse and randomly scattered with no evidence of nuclear localization. (Methyl green pyronin; magnification × 640; 34 days exposure.)

sites, it would not detract from the physiological significance of the findings, since nuclear type II sites have been shown to be related to uterotrophic response and are found predominantly in target organs.[22,23]

These studies also demonstrated the need for measures to decrease nonspecific binding in procedures involving the in vitro incubation of steroids with tissue slices. With in vivo studies, nonspecific binding is not often a problem because free and loosely bound estradiol is cleared by the blood while target cells retain the radioligand,[24] an important characteristic of these cells.[25] In early in vitro experiments without chase, however, the nonspecific binding over cellular and acellular areas was prohibitively high, hindering the identification of putative target cells. To decrease this background, a chase containing albumin in the medium was added to the method. Strobl et al.[26,27] have shown that the use of an albumin wash is more effective than medium only for decreasing bound estrogen and will also decrease specific binding to some extent. The albumin chase, while facilitating the identification of target cells, may, therefore, result in a possible decrease of sensitivity of the method. Nevertheless, it would appear that with in vitro experiments the use of a wash may be beneficial when the nonspecific binding is prohibitively high. For instance, Shannon et al.[19] used a chase with saline only, while in certain experiments Martin and Sheridan[5] employed an antiestradiol antibody wash.

## B. Human Tissue
### 1. Benign Lesions

Breast biopsies of 17 cases of benign mammary lesions were studied.[12] In four of nine fibroadenomas there was evidence of specific binding in ducts randomly scattered throughout the section and adjacent to other positive or negative ducts (Figure 3). On closer examination

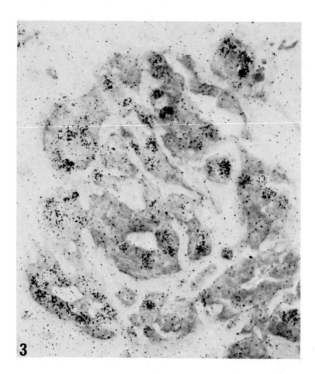

FIGURE 3.    Section of human fibroadenoma after in vitro incubation with ³H-estradiol only. Specific labeling is present in the nuclear region of many, but not all, epithelial cells of some ducts. (Hematoxylin and eosin; magnification × 400; 128 days exposure.)

the specific labeling was seen to be confined to the nuclear region of epithelial cells, while histologically identifiable myoepithelial cells were negative. In positive ducts labeled epithelial cells were admixed with negative cells. Stromal cells were generally unlabeled. In the negative cases, there were no areas where specific uptake could be identified, and sections of tissue incubated only in ³H-estradiol resembled those incubated with excess unlabeled estradiol or DES. The few randomly scattered grains revealed no evidence of a predominantly nuclear localization. In fibrocystic disease, specific uptake was identified in three of eight cases and the distribution of the specific labeling resembled that seen in fibroadenomas.

Biochemical assay of these lesions was not done and, thus, a direct comparison was not possible. In this survey of benign lesions, however, the relative percentage of positive and negative cases is similar to that published by others using biochemical assays as previously discussed.[12]

We found that myoepithelial and stromal cells were generally negative. The absence of specific labeling in myoepithelial cells agrees with the observation of Sar and Stumpf[17] on the lactating breast of experimental animals. These investigators[17] and others[50] also noted specific binding in some stromal cells in experimental animals, however, that was only very rarely observed in the human biopsies examined. This apparent discrepancy may be related to such factors as differences in techniques or differences in species and functional state.

*2. Malignant Lesions*

The distribution of ³H-estradiol uptake and retention was assessed in 40 cases of human breast cancer.[13,14] In the positive cases uptake was identified in some but not all of the neoplastic epithelial cells and could be suppressed by radioinert estradiol or DES (Figure 4). At high power grains were noted predominantly over the nuclear region, with relatively little cytoplasmic labeling (Figure 5). In nests of infiltrating tumor, labeled cells were admixed with unlabeled cells. The average number of nuclear grains per 10 $\mu m^2$ cross-sectional area in positive cells varied considerably.[13] The percentage of positive cells also seemed to vary from area to area over the slide but positive cells were seen in most regions.

The retention of radioactivity was restricted primarily to the neoplastic epithelial cells. Stromal cells were essentially negative with only an occasional cell showing nuclear labeling. In several cases, however, atypical hyperplasia as well as benign cysts were included within the tissue studied, and these lesions revealed, in some instances, positive epithelial cells intermingled with negative cells.[13] In several cases, foci of intraductal carcinoma within infiltrating lesions were evaluated.[14] These intraductal carcinomas showed a heterogeneous population of positive and negative cells in some areas (Figure 6), while elsewhere they were negative.

Negative tumors revealed no specific labeling and the appearances were similar to those of tissue incubated in excess radioinert estradiol or DES. The grains were sparse and randomly scattered throughout the field, with no tendency toward nuclear localization.

Of the 40 cases assessed autoradiographically, 31 (78%) were positive and 9 (22%) were negative. Thirty-seven cases were evaluated biochemically and 28 (76%) were positive, 6 (16%) borderline, and 3 (8%) negative.[13,14] A comparison of autoradiographic with biochemical data[13,14] revealed agreement in 26 of the 28 biochemically positive cases (93%) and all three of the negative cases. There were no autoradiographic criteria defined for borderline cases. For these cases[14] one was judged markedly positive autoradiographically, one weakly positive, and four negative. It was evident from this comparison that, in general, the autoradiographic method failed to detect specific binding of less than about 15 fmol/mg protein.[14]

These studies have clearly demonstrated that, as assessed by the present autoradiographic method, estrogen receptor-positive human mammary carcinomas are composed of a heterogenous population of target and nontarget cells. Such heterogeneity has been reported by others using immunocytochemical and histochemical methods[28-37] and has been suggested from biochemical[38,39] and clinical data.[40,41] The effect of this apparent heterogeneity on endocrine responsiveness of mammary carcinoma is not clear and requires more extensive investigation.

Stoll[42] has suggested that for a measurable response to endocrine therapy to occur, the requisite 50% decrease in tumor diameter necessitates a kill of 99% of the tumor cells. In this series of cases none were observed to contain 99% positive cells. It must be remembered, however, that in a morphologic assay such as this the tissue is examined at one point in time, and it is impossible to detect any modulation of ER within the cells over time. Moreover, since the positive target cells have been identified by their ability to bind $^3$H-estradiol as assessed by the number of nuclear grains, it may be that, at the time of examination, the nuclear receptor was inactivated, perhaps through the effects of a nuclear phosphatase[43] or estrogen receptor regulatory factor[44] as has been described in the uterus of experimental animals, or as part of the nuclear processing of ER as discussed by Horwitz and McGuire.[45]

In these experiments several areas of intraductal carcinoma were observed. Some were found to be positive while others were negative. This limited sample would suggest that the cell population of an intraductal lesion can be either ER-positive or -negative and would not support the suggestion of Lee[30] that intraductal areas are generally ER-negative. The number of areas sampled in the present investigation was limited, and further studies would be required to draw definite conclusions. A biochemical assessment of intraductal lesions,[46] however, has demonstrated a slightly greater proportion of positive cases than was found with infiltrating ductal lesions. The biochemical assay of intraductal lesions could, however,

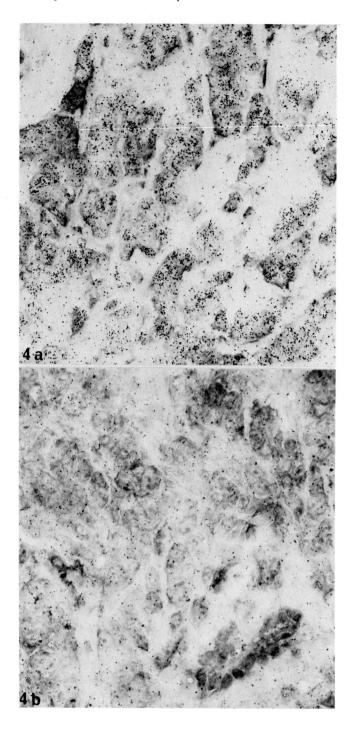

FIGURE 4.    (a) Section of estrogen receptor-positive human mammary carcinoma after in vitro incubation with ³H-estradiol only. The autoradiograph demonstrates the presence of specific labeling associated with many of the neoplastic epithelial cells. Closer examination revealed this label was located mainly over the nuclear region. (Hematoxylin and eosin; magnification × 400; 68 days exposure.) (b) Breast cancer tissue adjacent to that illustrated in Figure 4a after in vitro incubation with ³H-estradiol and a 100-fold excess of radioinert estradiol. The labeling seen is sparse with no evidence of a nuclear concentration. (Hematoxylin and eosin; magnification × 400; 68 days exposure.)

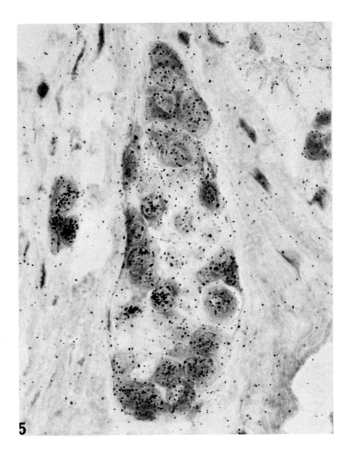

FIGURE 5.    High-power view of an estrogen receptor-positive infiltrating duct carcinoma incubated in $^3$H-estradiol only. This figure illustrates the predominantly nuclear localization of radioactivity in putative target cells admixed with unlabeled cells. The variability in degree of labeling among target cells is also apparent. (Hematoxylin and eosin; magnification × 600; 78 days exposure.)

be complicated by the inclusion of associated atypical hyperplastic lesions that, as described in this report, can be ER-positive, possibly resulting in a false biochemical assessment of these lesions.

In these studies, as with mouse uterus, the contribution to the labeling due to nuclear type II sites has not been evaluated. It is assumed that, like the uterus, these sites would have physiological significance but further studies would be necessary. It should be pointed out, however, that these sites can be correlated with the presence of cytoplasmic progesterone receptors, known to be a valuable indicator of patient response.[47]

The inability of the present method to detect positive cases with relatively low ER levels may result from possible loss of specific binding during the wash in medium with albumin as discussed earlier. Other possible factors include latent image fading and insufficient length of exposure. Another factor to be considered is negative chemography;[48] however, control studies done in several cases to assess this phenomenon revealed no evidence of decreased sensitivity of the photographic emulsion resulting from interaction with the tissue.

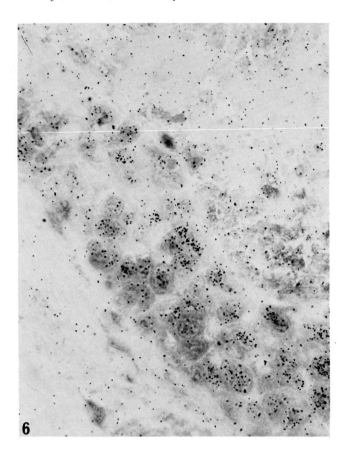

FIGURE 6.   An area of intraductal carcinoma from an estrogen receptor-positive infiltrating lesion. Some, but not all, neoplastic cells within this area reveal specific labeling. (Hematoxylin and eosin; magnification × 600; 66 days exposure.)

## IV. CONCLUSION

This report presents our findings concerning the distribution of putative estrogen target cells in human breast lesions using thaw-mount autoradiography as a means of localizing ³H-estradiol after in vitro incubation. As noted, dry-mount and thaw-mount autoradiography are accurate means of localizing steroid hormone binding sites in experimental animals. The necessity of in vitro incubation for the application of such methods to the study of human lesions introduces the potential for artifacts.[48] The results of these experiments indicate, however, that it is feasible to identify estrogen target cells in human tissue using these techniques.

In the development of morphologic methods applicable to the routine clinical evaluation of steroid hormone receptors in breast carcinoma, it is of paramount importance that consideration be given to established fundamental biochemical information. With morphologic methods employing protein-ligand interactions as a means of localizing receptors, it is difficult to determine essential parameters of the reaction such as affinity,[49] and one must rely on other criteria, including hormone specificity and appropriate target organ distribution. Correlative biochemical investigations to demonstrate the affinity of the ligand for receptor and other binding sites are also required. Most of this information is available in the case of thaw-mount autoradiography using ³H-estradiol as a ligand.[9] While other methods may well be able to predict therapeutic efficacy,[33] until the necessary basic research has been completed great care must be exercised in interpreting the data at the fundamental level. On the other hand, the autoradiographic method described here, while not readily adaptable to the clinical setting, may well serve as an investigative tool.

The data presented here and by others clearly suggest that human breast lesions contain a heterogeneous population of positive and negative cells. It is apparent, moreover, that a valid method for localizing steroid hormone receptors in breast cancer could supplement, if not replace, biochemical assays. These methods could provide information not readily obtained from biochemical assays, such as the receptor content of atypical hyperplasia and intraductal carcinoma in their evolution to frankly invasive carcinomas, and the relationship, if any, between the percent of receptor-containing cells and therapeutic efficacy. There is, therefore, a definite need for additional work in this field.

# REFERENCES

1. **Edwards, D. P., Chamness, G. C., and McGuire, W. L.,** Estrogen and progesterone receptor proteins in breast cancer, *Biochim. Biophys. Acta,* 560, 457, 1979.
2. **Stumpf, W. E. and Roth, L. J.,** High resolution autoradiography with dry mounted, freeze-dried frozen sections: comparative study of six methods using two diffusible compounds ³H-estradiol and ³H-mesobilirubinogen, *J. Histochem. Cytochem.,* 14, 274, 1966.
3. **Jensen, E. V., Suzuki, T., Kawashima, T., Stumpf, W. E., Jungblut, P. W., and DeSombre, E. R.,** A two-step mechanism for the interaction of estradiol with rat uterus, *Proc. Natl. Acad. Sci. U.S.A.,* 59, 632, 1968.
4. **Sheridan, P. J., Buchanan, J. M., Anselmo, V. C., and Martin, P. M.,** Equilibrium: the intracellular distribution of steroid receptors, *Nature (London),* 282, 579, 1979.
5. **Martin, P. M. and Sheridan, P. J.,** Towards a new model for the mechanism of action of steroids, *J. Steroid Biochem.,* 16, 215, 1982.
6. **Stumpf, W. E.,** Localization of hormones by autoradiography and other histochemical techniques. A critical review, *J. Histochem. Cytochem.,* 18, 21, 1970.
7. **Stumpf, W. E. and Sar, M.,** Autoradiographic localization of estrogen, androgen, progestin, and glucocorticosteroid in "target tissues" and "nontarget tissues", in *Receptors and Mechanism of Action of Steroid Hormones. Part I. Modern Pharmacology-Toxicology,* Vol. 8, Pasqualini, J. R., Ed., Marcel Dekker, New York, 1977, 41.
8. **Stumpf, W. E., Sar, M., Zuber, T. J., Soini, E., and Tuohimaa, P.,** Quantitative assessment of steroid hormone binding sites by thaw-mount autoradiography, *J. Histochem. Cytochem.,* 29, 201, 1981.
9. **Cunha, G. R., Shannon, J. M., Vanderslice, K. D., McCormick, K., and Bigsby, R. M.,** Autoradiographic demonstration of high affinity nuclear binding and finite binding capacity of [³H]estradiol in mouse vaginal cells, *Endocrinology,* 113, 1427, 1983.
10. **Cunha, G. R., Chung, L. W. K., Shannon, J. M., Taguchi, O., and Fujii, H.,** Hormone-induced morphogenesis and growth: role of mesenchymal-epithelial interactions, *Recent Prog. Horm. Res.,* 39, 559, 1983.
11. **Buell, R. H. and Tremblay, G.,** Autoradiographic demonstration of uptake and retention of ³H-estradiol after in vitro incubation, *J. Histochem. Cytochem.,* 29, 1316, 1981.
12. **Buell, R. H. and Tremblay, G.,** Autoradiographic demonstration of ³H-estradiol incorporation in benign human mammary lesions, *Am. J. Clin. Pathol.,* 81, 30, 1984.
13. **Buell, R. H. and Tremblay, G.,** The localization of ³H-estradiol in estrogen receptor-positive human mammary carcinoma as visualized by thaw-mount autoradiography, *Cancer,* 51, 1625, 1983.
14. **Buell, R. H. and Tremblay, G.,** in preparation.
15. **Puca, G. A. and Bresciani, F.,** Interactions of 6,7-³H-17β-estradiol with mammary gland and other organs of the C3H mouse *in vivo, Endocrinology,* 85, 1, 1969.
16. **McGuire, W. L. and DeLaGarza, M.,** Improved sensitivity in the measurement of estrogen receptor in human breast cancer, *J. Clin. Endocrinol. Metab.,* 37, 986, 1973.

17. **Sar, M. and Stumpf, W. E.,** Autoradiography of mammary glands and uteri of mice and rats after the injection of [$^3$H]-estradiol, *J. Steroid Biochem.,* 7, 391, 1976.

18. **Gorski, J., Toft, D., Shyamala, G., Smith, D., and Notides, A.,** Hormone receptors: studies on the interaction of estrogen with the uterus, *Recent Prog. Horm. Res.,* 24, 45, 1968.

19. **Shannon, J. M., Cunha, G. R., Taguchi, O., Vanderslice, K. D., and Gould, S. F.,** Autoradiographic localization of steroid binding in human tissue labeled in vitro, *J. Histochem. Cytochem.,* 30, 1059, 1982.

20. **Eriksson, H., Upchurch, S., Hardin, J. W., Peck, E. J., Jr., and Clark, J. H.,** Heterogeneity of estrogen receptors in the cytosol and nuclear fractions of the rat uterus, *Biochem. Biophys. Res. Commun.,* 81, 1, 1978.

21. **Clark, J. H., Hardin, J. W., Upchurch, S., and Eriksson, H.,** Heterogeneity of estrogen binding sites in the cytosol of the rat uterus, *J. Biol. Chem.,* 253, 7630, 1978.

22. **Eriksson, H. A., Hardin, J. W., Markaverich, B., Upchurch, S., and Clark, J. H.,** Estrogen binding in the rat uterus: heterogeneity of sites and relation to uterotrophic response, *J. Steroid Biochem.,* 12, 121, 1980.

23. **Markaverich, B. M., Upchurch, S., and Clark, J. H.,** Two binding sites for estradiol in rat uterine nuclei: relationship to stimulation and antagonism of uterine growth, in *Perspectives in Steroid Receptor Research,* Bresciani, F., Ed., Raven Press, New York, 1980, 143.

24. **Jensen, E. V. and Jacobson, H. I.,** Fate of steroid estrogens in target tissues, in *Biological Activities of Steroids in Relation to Cancer,* Pincus, G. and Vollmer, E. P., Eds., Academic Press, New York, 1960, 161.

25. **Katzenellenbogen, B. S.,** Dynamics of steroid hormone receptor action, *Annu. Rev. Physiol.,* 42, 17, 1980.

26. **Strobl, J. S. and Lippman, M. E.,** Prolonged retention of estradiol by human breast cancer cells in tissue culture, *Cancer Res.,* 39, 3319, 1979.

27. **Strobl, J. S., Monaco, M. E., and Lippman, M. E.,** The role of intracellular equilibria and the effect of antiestrogens on estrogen-receptor dissociation kinetics from perfused cultures of human breast cancer cells, *Endocrinology,* 107, 450, 1980.

28. **Lee, S. H.,** Cytochemical study of estrogen receptor in human mammary cancer, *Am. J. Clin. Pathol.,* 70, 197, 1978.

29. **Lee, S. H.,** Cellular estrogen and progesterone receptors in mammary carcinoma, *Am. J. Clin. Pathol.,* 73, 323, 1980.

30. **Lee, S. H.,** Cancer cell estrogen receptor of human mammary carcinoma, *Cancer,* 44, 1, 1979.

31. **Pertschuk, L. P., Tobin, E. H., Brigati, D. J., Kim, D. S., Bloom, N. D., Gaetjens, E., Berman, P. J., Carter, A. C., and Degenshein, G. A.,** Immunofluorescent detection of estrogen receptors in breast cancer. Comparison with dextran-coated charcoal and sucrose gradient assays, *Cancer,* 41, 907, 1978.

32. **Pertschuk, L. P., Gaetjens, E., Carter, A. C., Brigati, D. J., Kim, D. S., and Fealey, T. E.,** An improved histochemical method for detection of estrogen receptors in mammary cancer. Comparison with biochemical assay, *Am. J. Clin. Pathol.,* 71, 504, 1979.

33. **Pertschuk, L. P., Tobin, E. H., Gaetjens, E., Carter, A. C., Degenshein, G. A., Bloom, N. D., and Brigati, D. J.,** Histochemical assay of estrogen and progesterone receptors in breast cancer: correlation with biochemical assays and patients' response to endocrine therapies, *Cancer,* 46, 2896, 1980.

34. **Pertschuk, L. P., Tobin, E. H., Brigati, D. J., and Gaetjens, E.,** Morphologic assay of steroid hormone receptors in human neoplasia, *Pathol. Annu.,* 15 (Part 2), 143, 1980.

35. **Hanna, W., Ryder, D. E., and Mobbs, B. G.,** Cellular localization of estrogen binding sites in human breast cancer, *Am. J. Clin. Pathol.,* 77, 391, 1982.

36. **Fisher, B., Gunduz, N., Zheng, S., and Saffer, E. A.,** Fluoresceinated estrone binding by human and mouse breast cancer cells, *Cancer Res.,* 42, 540, 1982.

37. **Barrows, G. H., Stroupe, S. B., and Riehm, J. D.,** Nuclear uptake of a 17β-estradiol-fluorescein derivative as a marker of estrogen dependence, *Am. J. Clin. Pathol.,* 73, 330, 1980.

38. **Børjesson, B. W. and Sarfaty, G. A.,** Estradiol receptors in subpopulations of breast cancer cells isolated from human primary tumors, *Cancer,* 47, 1828, 1981.

39. **Rao, B. R. and Meyer, J. S.,** Estrogen and progestin receptors in normal and cancer tissue, in *Progress in Cancer Research and Therapy, Vol. 4, Progesterone Receptors in Normal and Neoplastic Tissues,* McGuire, W. L., Raynaud, J.-P., and Baulieu, E.-E., Eds., Raven Press, New York, 1977, 155.

40. **Rosen, P. P., Menendez-Botet, C. J., Urban, J. A., Fracchia, A., and Schwartz, M. K.,** Estrogen receptor protein (ERP) in multiple tumor specimens from individual patients with breast cancer, *Cancer,* 39, 2194, 1977.

41. **Allegra, J. C., Barlock, A., Huff, K. K., and Lippman, M. E.,** Changes in multiple or sequential estrogen receptor determinations in breast cancer, *Cancer,* 45, 792, 1980.

42. **Stoll, B. A.,** ''False-positive'' oestrogen-receptor assay in breast cancer, *Lancet,* 2, 296, 1977.

43. **Auricchio, F., Migliaccio, A., Castoria, G., Lastoria, S., and Rotondi, A.,** Evidence that *in vivo* estradiol receptor translocated into nuclei is dephosphorylated and released into cytoplasm, *Biochem. Biophys. Res. Commun.,* 106, 149, 1982.
44. **Okulicz, W. C., Evans, R. W., and Leavitt, W. W.,** Progesterone regulation of the occupied form of nuclear estrogen receptor, *Science,* 213, 1503, 1981.
45. **Horwitz, K. B. and McGuire, W. L.,** Nuclear mechanisms of estrogen action: effects of estradiol and anti-estrogens on estrogen receptors and nuclear receptor processing, *J. Biol. Chem.,* 253, 8185, 1978.
46. **McCarty, K. S., Jr., Barton, T. K., Fetter, B. F., Woodard, B. H., Mossler, J. A., Reeves, W., Daly, J., Wilkinson, W. E., and McCarty, K. S., Sr.,** Correlation of estrogen and progesterone receptors with histologic differentiation in mammary carcinoma, *Cancer,* 46, 2851, 1980.
47. **Syne, J. S., Markaverich, B. M., Clark, J. H., and Panko, W. B.,** Estrogen binding sites in the nucleus of normal and malignant human tissue: characteristics of the multiple nuclear binding sites, *Cancer Res.,* 42, 4449, 1982.
48. **Stumpf, W. E.,** High-resolution autoradiography and its application to *in vitro* experiments: subcellular localization of ³H-estradiol in rat uterus, in *Radioisotopes in Medicine: In Vitro Studies,* Symp. Series 13, Hayes, R. L., Goswitz, F. A., and Murphy, G., Eds., Atomic Energy Commission, Oak Ridge, Tenn., 1968, 633.
49. **Morrow, B., Leav, I., DeLellis, R. A., and Raam, S.,** Use of polyestradiol phosphate and anti-17β estradiol antibodies for the localization of estrogen receptors in target tissues: a critique, *Cancer,* 46, 2872, 1980.
50. **Buell, R. H. and Tremblay, G.,** unpublished observation.

Chapter 2

# MORPHOLOGIC DETECTION OF MULTIPLE STEROID BINDING SITES IN BREAST CANCER BY HISTOCHEMISTRY AND BY IMMUNOCYTOCHEMISTRY WITH MONOCLONAL ANTIRECEPTOR ANTIBODY: RELATIONSHIP TO ENDOCRINE RESPONSE*

**Louis P. Pertschuk, Karen B. Eisenberg, Anne C. Carter, and Joseph G. Feldman**

## TABLE OF CONTENTS

I.      Introduction ................................................................... 16

II.    Comparison of Two Different Histochemical Estrogen Binding Methods ........ 16
      A.     Methodology ......................................................... 16
      B.     Comparison of Results of 6-FE and 17-FE ............................. 17
      C.     Comparison of 6-FE, 17-FE, and DCC .................................. 17

III.   Estrogen Receptor Immunocytochemical Assay (ERICA) ....................... 21
      A.     Method ............................................................... 21
      B.     Results of ERICA: Comparison with DCC, 6-FE, and 17-FE ............ 21
      C.     The Apparent Nuclear Location of ER by ERICA ...................... 21

IV.   Clinical Correlations ....................................................... 25
      A.     Single and Combined Methodologies in 32 Breast Cancer Patients: Clinical
             Correlations ....................................................... 25
      B.     Clinical Correlation with 17-FE and DCC ............................ 27
      C.     Clinical Correlation with the Addition of Progesterone Binding Data .... 28
      D.     ER and PgR by Biochemical Assay: Clinical Correlations ............... 28
      E.     EB and PB by Histochemistry: Clinical Correlations .................... 29
      F.     Combined ER, PgR, EB, and PB Assay Results: Clinical Correlations .. 29
      G.     Other Histochemical-Clinical Correlations ............................. 30

V.     Differences between 6-FE and 17-FE ......................................... 30

VI.    Nuclear Binding of 17-FE ................................................... 33

Acknowledgments ................................................................. 33

References ....................................................................... 33

* Supported by USPHS Grant No. CA23623 from NCI.

# I. INTRODUCTION

There is general agreement that a valid histologic method for detection of steroid receptors in human breast cancer would be a valuable clinical tool.[1] Such a technique would allow oncologists at the community hospital level to select rational treatment for patients with advanced, metastatic disease. Furthermore, by permitting determinations of tumor cell steroid binding heterogeneity and allowing for evaluation of the potential contribution of nonmalignant tissue elements to the total steroid binding capacity of a specimen, a histologic procedure would be an important adjunct to conventional biochemical receptor assays. The latter, performed on fractions obtained by ultracentrifugation of tissue homogenates, do not permit such assessments.

Although a number of different methods designed to detect estrogen receptor (ER) have been reported, none have been unequivocally shown to detect the classical type I ER ordinarily measured biochemically. On the contrary, they have been the subjects of considerable criticism.[2-4] These criticisms are based upon two main points: (1) histologic assays employ a concentration of binding ligand in excess of that required to saturate type I ER in biochemical systems, as well as an excess of competitor ligands for displacement; and (2) it is questioned whether such methods are capable of visualizing the finite number of receptors estimated to be present in the average cancer cell. In a recent review of this subject[5] we arrived at the following conclusions. Information as to binding kinetics obtained by biochemical assay may not be directly applicable to a histochemical system. Consequently, histologic methods might, indeed, be detecting type I ER which might behave differently in a histologic rather than a biochemical milieu. On the other hand, these methods might be detecting type II and/or type III binding sites as well as organelle or membrane-bound ER.

The development of monoclonal antibodies specific for type I ER by Greene and colleagues[6,7] and the creation of an estrogen receptor immunocytochemical assay (ERICA) by this group[8,9] has afforded the opportunity to compare results of other histochemical techniques with this entirely new approach and, thus, perhaps, to gain additional insight into the nature of the binding revealed by these procedures.

# II. COMPARISON OF TWO DIFFERENT HISTOCHEMICAL ESTROGEN BINDING METHODS

## A. Methodology

We compared results of estrogen binding (EB) by the method of Lee[10] employing 17-beta-estradiol-6-*O*-carboxymethyloxime-bovine serum albumin-fluorescein isothiocyanate (6-FE) with that of Pertschuk et al.[11] The latter, developed in our laboratory, utilized 17-beta-estradiol-17-hemisuccinyl-bovine serum albumin-fluorescein isothiocyanate (17-FE) as the binding ligand.

Breast cancer specimens from 173 patients were studied and the results compared to ER by the dextran-coated charcoal assay (DCC) performed in the majority of cases in the laboratory of Dr. William L. McGuire at the University of Texas Health Sciences Center at San Antonio. Results of DCC were not available at the time of histochemical assay.

Specimens for 6-FE were processed as outlined by Lee.[10] Frozen tissue sections were rehydrated in phosphate buffered saline (PBS) containing bovine serum albumin (BSA) and then incubated for 2 hr at 24°C with $2 \times 10^{-4}$ $M$ of ligand. The sections were then washed in buffer. For 17-FE, frozen tumor sections were exposed to $7 \times 10^{-7}$ $M$ of ligand diluted in PBS, containing 10% ethanol, for 2 hr at 24°C, postfixed in acetone-ethanol, and then washed in buffer.

In order to allow for comparison of assay results we used the following criteria for interpretation. A specimen was considered as positive for 6-FE when 10% or more of the component tumor cells showed a level of fluorescent intensity rated as $+2$. A specimen was classified as positive for 17-FE when 10% or more of the tumor cells exhibited a fluorescent intensity judged to be +1. This difference was necessary as 6-FE contained more moles of fluorescein per mole BAS than did 17-FE. For DCC, specimens containing more than 10 fmol/mg protein were considered as positive.

## B. Comparison of Results of 6-FE and 17-FE

It was obvious that there were differences in the binding of 6-FE and 17-FE. There were specimens clearly positive with 6-FE which were 17-FE-negative, while the converse situation also occurred. In addition, even when both assays were qualitatively positive, tumors were encountered in which it was quite apparent that different cell populations were binding each ligand. There were also specimens where 17-FE resulted in nuclear binding, whereas binding of 6-FE was cytoplasmic, and others where 17-FE resulted in nucleolar binding which was not observed with 6-FE. Some of these differences in binding of 6-FE and 17-FE are illustrated in Figures 1 and 2.

Despite these differences, when the overall results were compared (Table 1) there was basic agreement as to positivity or negativity in 66%. Using the Kappa statistic (K) to evaluate the level of agreement between methods (K = 1 = perfect agreement; K = 0 = no agreement), it was found that the level of agreement was only fair (K = 0.323). However, there was a statistical clear association between the two methods unlikely to be due to chance alone ($p$ <0.001).

## C. Comparison of 6-FE, 17-FE, and DCC

Comparison of results of 6-FE and DCC revealed agreement in 64% of the 173 cases (Table 2). Similar findings were obtained when results of 17-FE were correlated with DCC results. There was concordance in 68% (Table 3). Statistical analyses of these data again showed that there was a significant association between all the methods ($p$ <0.001) but with only a fair level of agreement (K = 0.284 for 6-FE and DCC; K = 0.278 for 17-FE and DCC).

These results were not dissimilar to those previously published. Earlier, Hasson[12] had studied a series of breast cancers with 6-FE and 17-FE and had noted some discrepancies. Bohm et al.[13] had not apparently observed any discrepancy between these two ligands in an analysis of 70 breast cancer specimens.

Numerous workers have compared results of 6-FE with those of DCC with degrees of concordance ranging from 62 to 90%. Jacobs et al.[14] obtained agreement in 63% of 48 cases, Alonso and Brownlee[15] in 67% of 21 cases, Tominaga and co-workers[16] in 76% of 50 cases, Hanna et al.[17] in 62% of 34 cases, Hasson[12] in 66% of 101 cases, and Bohm et al.[13] in 90% of 70 cases. Meijer et al.[18] were also able to successfully correlate results in 90% of 132 cases. Berger and colleagues[19] obtained good agreement in 86% of 14 cases, O'Connell and Said[20] in 85% of 26 specimens, while Panko et al.[21] only correlated results successfully in 63% of 49 cases. It is difficult to evaluate the results obtained by Sismondi et al.[22] In their abstract they merely state that there was no correlation between 6-FE and DCC in 839 cases.

Fewer investigators have had the opportunity to compare results of 17-FE and DCC, as 17-FE is not commercially available. Hasson[12] obtained satisfactory concordance in 65% of 68 cases, Bohm et al.[13] in 90% of 70 cases, and Davis and co-workers[23] in 87% of 38 cases.

The causes for the wide variations in reported agreement, i.e., 62 to 90% of 6-FE and 65 to 90% of 17-FE, are not readily apparent. We have pointed out several reasons why histochemical and biochemical results may not always concur,[11] even assuming that they are both a measure of the same estrogen binding site. This may occur when specimens contain relatively few tumor cells and a large amount of stroma or when a specimen is extremely cellular. In such instances, the amount of receptor protein in the tumor cytosol may be diluted to a level where it is undetectable biochemically, or paradoxically contain biochemically measurable ER reflecting the sum total contribution of innumerable cells

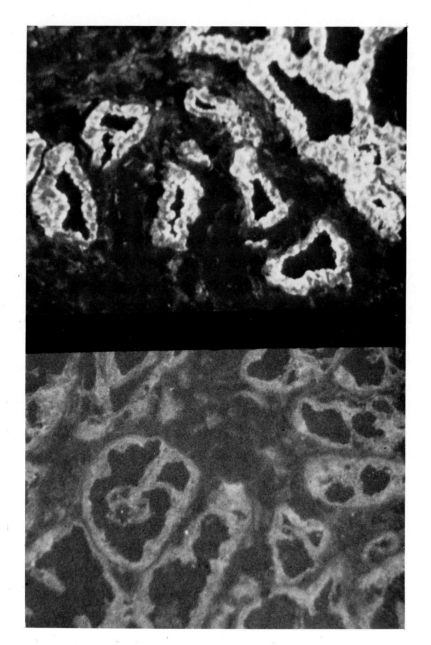

FIGURE 1. Well-differentiated adenocarcinoma of the breast. (A, left) Shows poor uptake of 17-FE ligand-conjugate; and (B, right) strongly positive cytoplasmic binding of 6-FE ligand. (Magnification × 100.)

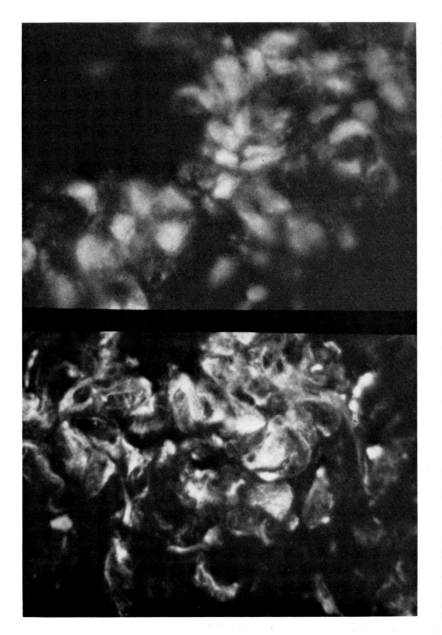

FIGURE 2. High-power view of mammary carcinoma showing heterogeneous uptake of cytoplasmic 6-FE (A, left) and nuclear binding of 17-FE (B, right). (Magnification × 500.)

### Table 1
### COMPARISON OF ESTROGEN BINDING WITH 6-FE AND 17-FE IN BREAST CANCER

|        | 17-FE + | 17-FE − | Total |
|--------|---------|---------|-------|
| 6-FE + | 70      | 15      | 85    |
| 6-FE − | 44      | 44      | 88    |
| Total  | 114     | 59      | 173   |

### Table 2
### COMPARISON OF ESTROGEN BINDING BY 6-FE WITH ER BY DCC IN BREAST CANCER

|       | 6-FE + | 6-FE − | Total |
|-------|--------|--------|-------|
| DCC + | 69     | 45     | 114   |
| DCC − | 17     | 42     | 59    |
| Total | 86     | 87     | 173   |

### Table 3
### COMPARISON OF ESTROGEN BINDING BY 17-FE WITH ER BY DCC IN BREAST CANCER

|       | 17-FE + | 17-FE − | Total |
|-------|---------|---------|-------|
| DCC + | 86      | 28      | 114   |
| DCC − | 28      | 31      | 59    |
| Total | 114     | 59      | 173   |

which, individually, may be very low in receptor content. Furthermore, since biochemical assays are performed on tumor cytosol, nuclear binding sites and binding sites on cell membranes or organelles may go undetected. Since different blocks of tumor are usually used for each assay, tissue heterogeneity may also be responsible for divergent results. It is conceivable that those workers reporting relatively low correlations made no allowance for any of these factors. Finally, if, indeed, biochemical and histochemical methods detect different but associated binding sites, then it would be anticipated that agreement between assay results would be imperfect.

In our present series of 173 cases we have not made any allowance for any of the above factors, since we no longer feel compelled to fit the histochemical with the biochemical data. Be that as it may, from a statistical viewpoint it is quite apparent that there is a significant association between EB studies with both 6-FE and 17-FE and ER by DCC in the hands of a number of different workers, beyond that which could be expected by chance, although the level of agreement is not perfect.

All of these data quite strongly suggest that the three assay systems, i.e., 6-FE, 17-FE, and DCC, are detecting estrogen binding sites that are significantly associated with each other, but which in all probability are actually different.

## III. ESTROGEN RECEPTOR IMMUNOCYTOCHEMICAL ASSAY (ERICA)

### A. Method

ERICA was performed in the following way according to the technique developed by G. Greene and W. King, University of Chicago. Frozen tissue sections were fixed in picric acid/paraformaldehyde, exposed to ovalbumin to reduce nonspecific binding, and then incubated with 40 to 80 $\mu\ell$ of pooled monoclonal antiestrophilin antibody per milliliter PBS. We used the D547 Sp$\gamma$ and D75Sp$\gamma$ antibodies of Dr. Greene. After exposure to the pool for 30 min, the sections were washed in PBS, reacted with goat anti-rat IgG (since the monoclonal antibody was of rat origin), and then with rat peroxidase antiperoxidase complex (PAP). The reaction product was made visible with diaminobenzidine tetrahydrochloride and $H_2O_2$ in the usual way. No counterstain was employed. For control sections, normal rat IgG was substituted for the monoclonal antibody pool, or the pool was eliminated entirely. In some experiments, specifically absorbed antibody, supplied by Dr. Greene, was used. Specimens were considered positive for ER when at least 10% of the component tumor cells exhibited staining. Cases (103) previously analyzed with 6-FE, 17-FE, and DCC were studied.

### B. Results of ERICA: Comparison with DCC, 6-FE, and 17-FE

Specimens positive with ERICA invariably showed nuclear staining (Figures 3 and 4). Controls were all satisfactory. Heterogeneity of staining was a commonly observed feature both as to percentage of positive cells and intensity of the staining reaction (Figure 4).

Comparison of ERICA and DCC is shown in Table 4. There was concordance in 87%. In addition to a statistical association beyond chance ($p < 0.001$) there was a very significant level of agreement (K = 0.73). It was clear that the binding site revealed by ERICA was entirely different from that revealed by 6-FE and 17-FE, if for no other reason than ERICA's invariable nuclear localization. The close agreement of ERICA with DCC suggested that the two assays were probably measuring the same specific binding site (type I ER).

Comparison of 6-FE, 17-FE, and ERICA again showed a degree of association beyond chance ($p < 0.001$) with K values indicative of only a fair level of agreement (K $\cong$ <0.30; data not shown).

### C. The Apparent Nuclear Location of ER by ERICA

The elegant studies of Greene and colleagues[6,7] leave little room for doubting that these monoclonal antibodies are specific for type I ER. The nuclear localization of ER was, therefore, somewhat surprising in view of current dogma stating that initial steroid binding to receptor occurs in the cytoplasm and the obvious fact that biochemical ER assay is performed on tumor cytosols. One possible explanation of this phenomenon is that while in the cytoplasm, the antigenic determinants on the receptor protein molecule recognized by these monoclonal antibodies are hidden. After translocation, the determinants are exposed and, thus, available to bind to antibody. Another possibility is that the initial fixation step required for ERICA itself induces nuclear translocation. It, also, may be that ER is really within the nucleus and it is possible that during the processing required for biochemical assay ER is extracted into the cytosol. A nuclear location for ER as revealed by ERICA is in conformance with several autoradiographic studies[24-26] as well as with some of the biochemical data.[27,28]

Earlier, we and others had reported a cytoplasmic location for ER using immunocytochemical methods with these same monoclonal antibodies. In our laboratory we had employed a biotin-avidin technique on frozen tissue sections and detected cytoplasmic staining.[29] We had also obtained quite satisfactory correlations with DCC. However, we later discovered that the bridging biotinylated anti-rat IgG required for this procedure was capable of non-

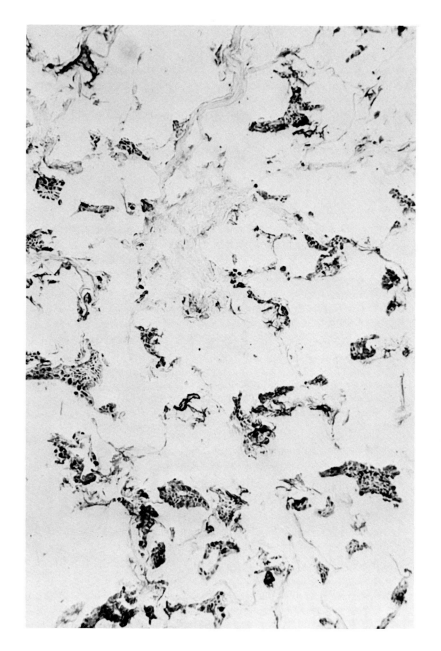

FIGURE 3.    Colloid carcinoma after staining with ERICA showing nuclear localization of receptor.  (Magnification  × 100.)

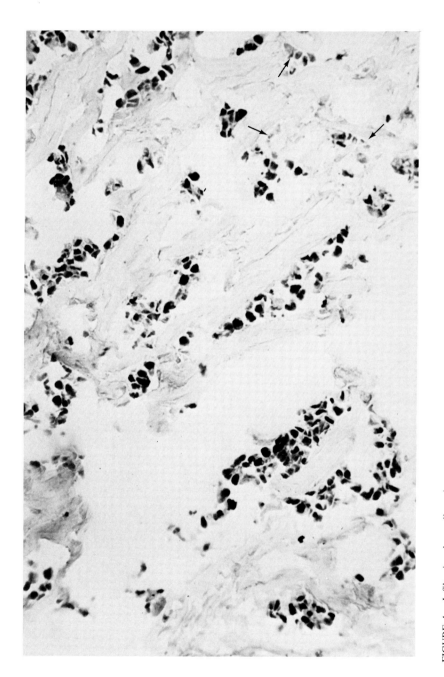

FIGURE 4. Infiltrating duct cell carcinoma processed by ERICA showing nuclear localization of receptor. Heterogeneity is evident, with some cells showing weak to no staining (arrows). (Magnification × 500.)

**Table 4**
## COMPARISON OF ERICA WITH
## ER BY DCC IN BREAST CANCER

|        | ERICA + | ERICA − | Total |
|--------|---------|---------|-------|
| DCC +  | 59      | 12      | 71    |
| DCC −  | 1       | 31      | 32    |
| Total  | 60      | 43      | 103   |

specific binding and, therefore, abandoned the method. Nadji and Morales[30] and Garancis and co-workers[31] employed a PAP method using paraffin-embedded tissue sections. They both reported a satisfactory level of correlation of cytoplasmic staining and biochemical ER assay. However, we have never been able to reproduce these results, and at this point in time it would appear that much of the cytoplasmic staining seen by these two groups was nonspecific.

The question now arises as to why there should be any correlation whatsoever between nonspecific cytoplasmic binding and ER by DCC. One logical conclusion is that functioning ER codes for multiple cytoplasmic proteins, some of which might possess avid nonspecific binding capacities. Tumors which lack ER would also lack these cytoplasmic proteins and fail to exhibit cytoplasmic staining, while those possessing ER could bind antibodies or other proteins in a nonspecific manner. To our knowledge, Nadji et al. have never demonstrated nuclear translocation by their technique, and we, also, were not able to demonstrate nuclear translocation with the biotin-avidin method. On the other hand, it is doubtful that the binding of 17-FE and 6-FE is of a nonspecific nature since it may be almost totally inhibited by specific competitors (17-FE) or blocked by preincubation with a steroid-BSA conjugate (6-FE).

Development of a valid immunohistologic ER technique eliminates many of the controversies surrounding the earlier methods. Immediate fixation of the tissue section prevents loss of soluble antigen, while the high sensitivity of the PAP procedure permits visualization of a finite number of receptor sites.

It is difficult to compare ERICA's nuclear location with the cytoplasmic staining reported by Raam and colleagues. The latter group employed a polyclonal antibody to receptor-rich cytosol.[32] They, also, were able to apparently demonstrate nuclear translocation.[33] The polyclonality of their serum, however, may enable detection of other binding sites not recognized by the monoclonal antibodies used in ERICA.

Greene and colleagues[7] have demonstrated that their monoclonal antibodies recognize occupied as well as unoccupied ER. This is of importance for specimens from premenopausal women where endogenous estradiol would be expected to occupy receptor and might prevent its detection by conventional means. They have also performed elegant immunocytochemical controls which are strongly supportive of the assumption that ERICA recognizes type I ER.[49] They prepared dilutions of antibody in cytosol derived from the MCF-7 human breast cancer cell line which was known to be ER-positive. Similar dilutions of antibody were prepared in MCF-7 cytosol which had been depleted of ER by affinity chromatography or on an estradiol-Sepharose column. Additional dilutions were then made in depleted cytosol to which highly purified ER had been readded. In these experiments, specimens which were positive by ERICA became negative when reacted with ER-positive cytosol, positive in ER-depleted cytosol, and again negative when reacted with depleted cytosol plus ER. These experiments clearly demonstrate that the other cytoplasmic components, present in ER-positive cells, were unable to bind the monoclonal antibodies and are very convincing demonstrations of the antibodies' specificity for ER. On the other hand, Raam et al.[32]

adsorbed their polyclonal antibody only with receptor-rich cytosol. The negative staining which was then obtained may, thus, have been due to multiple cytoplasmic components besides ER competing for antibody.

In experiments employing similar monoclonal antibodies to those used in our laboratory, Greene and co-workers[6] found that the observed limiting dilutions showed excellent agreement with the concentration of estradiol expected to saturate type I ER, being on the order of 1.5 to 7.0 $\times$ $10^{-9}$ $M$.

## IV. CLINICAL CORRELATIONS

Of significantly greater importance than conformity with biochemical data both from a practical viewpoint as well as in helping to shed some light upon the nature of the binding revealed by histologic assays is their level of agreement with the clinical hormone responsiveness of breast cancer patients.

In an early study employing estrogen as the initial ligand and antiestrogen antibody and label for visualization, Mercer et al.[34] examined the relationship of tumor growth after ovariectomy to steroid binding homogeneity in rats. They showed that the extent of tumor regression correlated with the percentage of steroid binding cells. Furthermore, specimens which showed steroid binding before oophorectomy failed to evidence hormonal binding postsurgically. This interesting and provocative immunohistologic study and its possible relationship to human tumor endocrine response has not received the attention it rightfully deserves.

### A. Single and Combined Methodologies in 32 Breast Cancer Patients: Clinical Correlations

Among the cases which were analyzed by all four methodologies, i.e., 6-FE, 17-FE, ERICA, and DCC, were a group of 32 women with advanced metastatic breast carcinoma who had undergone endocrine treatment where the clinical response was known. We analyzed the response to hormonal therapy individually for each assay as well as by combined assay results for all systems (Tables 5 and 6). Criteria for positivity for each assay were the same as we have previously outlined.

There were 16 patients who were ERICA-positive; 14 (88%) of these women either responded to therapy or evidenced stabilization of their disease process. There were 16 patients who were ERICA-negative of whom 14 (88%) failed therapy. Thus, ERICA showed a specificity of 88% and a sensitivity of 88% where specificity is defined as the percentage of treatment failures with a negative assay and sensitivity as the percentage of responders (or women stabilized) with a positive assay.

There was insufficient tissue for DCC in one case. Of the remainder, 22 were DCC-positive. Fourteen (64%) either responded or became stable. There were 9 DCC-negative cases of whom 7 (78%) failed. Thus, the sensitivity of DCC was 88% and the specificity was 47%. Twenty-five women were 6-FE-positive. Fourteen (56%) either responded or became stable. Seven were 6-FE-negative of whom five failed therapy (71%). The sensitivity of 6-FE was 88% and the specificity was 31%. Twenty-five patients were 17-FE-positive (not the same exact patients as with 6-FE). Sixteen (64%) responded or were stabilized. Seven women were 17-FE-negative and all failed endocrine treatment. The sensitivity of 17-FE was 100% while the specificity was 44%.

Surprisingly, however, when all four of the assay results were positive as it was in 12 cases, the predictive value was the highest. All 12 of these women responded or became stable (100%). On the other hand, if any one assay was negative, the likelihood of a successful response was greatly diminished with 80% of these patients failing therapy. Statistical analyses of these data by both the Rank Sum and Chi square tests of trends and proportions

**Table 5**
## COMPARISON OF VARIOUS ESTROGEN BINDING ASSAYS IN BREAST CANCER WITH CLINICAL RESPONSE TO HORMONAL THERAPIES

(Series 1)

| Assay system | Result | Cases (#) | Failures (#) | Responding or stable (#) |
|---|---|---|---|---|
| ERICA | + | 16 | 2 | 14 |
| | − | 16 | 14 | 2 |
| 6-FE | + | 25 | 11 | 14 |
| | − | 7 | 5 | 2 |
| 17-FE | + | 25 | 9 | 16 |
| | − | 7 | 7 | 0 |
| DCC[a] | + | 22 | 8 | 14 |
| | − | 9 | 7 | 2 |

[a] One case not assayed by DCC.

**Table 6**
## COMBINED ESTROGEN BINDING ASSAY RESULTS: RELATIONSHIP TO ENDOCRINE RESPONSE

(Series 1)

| Type of assay and results | | | | Cases (#) | Failing (#) | Responding (#) | Stable (#) |
|---|---|---|---|---|---|---|---|
| 17-FE | 6-FE | ERICA | DCC | | | | |
| + | + | + | + | 12 | 0 | 9 | 3 |
| − | − | − | − | 2 | 2 | 0 | 0 |
| + | + | − | − | 4 | 2 | 2 | 0 |
| + | + | − | + | 4 | 4 | 0 | 0 |
| + | − | − | + | 1 | 1 | 0 | 0 |
| + | − | + | + | 3 | 1 | 2 | 0 |
| − | + | + | + | 1 | 1 | 0 | 0 |
| − | + | − | + | 1 | 1 | 0 | 0 |
| − | + | − | − | 3 | 3 | 0 | 0 |
| + | − | − | Not done | 1 | 1 | 0 | 0 |

showed that it was highly unlikely that these findings were solely due to chance ($p < 0.001$). The predictive value of the combined results for a successful response to hormonal treatment when all were positive was 100%, whereas the predictive value for treatment failure if any one test was negative was 80%. The sensitivity of the combined assay systems was 75% with a specificity of 100%.

All of the above data, together with the experimental work to be discussed a little later, support the hypothesis that 6-FE and 17-FE recognize two different estrogen binding sites. These binding loci are usually in the cytoplasm for 6-FE and in cytoplasm, nucleus, or nucleolus for 17-FE. These two binding sites are not only associated with each other but with a third site, detected in the nucleus by ERICA, and possibly extracted into and measured in the cytosol by DCC. In addition, there appears to exist a degree of positive cooperativity among the binding sites so that in order for tumor hormone response to be optimal, all must

**Table 7**
**COMPARISON OF RESULTS OF ESTROGEN**
**BINDING BY 17-FE WITH ENDOCRINE**
**RESPONSE IN BREAST CANCER**

(Series 2)

| Assay results | Cases (#) | Failed (#) | Responded (#) | Stable (#) |
|---|---|---|---|---|
| Positive | 72 | 31 | 39 | 2 |
| Negative | 48 | 44 | 3 | 1 |
| Nuclear binding | 30 | 23 | 7 | 0 |

**Table 8**
**COMPARISON OF RESULTS OF ER BY**
**DCC WITH ENDOCRINE RESPONSE IN**
**BREAST CANCER**

(Series 2)

| Assay results | Cases (#) | Failed (#) | Responded (#) | Stable (#) |
|---|---|---|---|---|
| Positive | 107 | 60 | 44 | 3 |
| Negative | 37 | 34 | 3 | 0 |

be present. Moreover, the absence of any one of these sites makes it unlikely that there will be an endocrine response.

The existence of multiple estrogen binding sites has already been shown by biochemical procedures,[35,36] and in breast cancer, a close association has been shown to exist between sites.[37] Clark and colleagues, in summarizing knowledge of estrogen binding site heterogeneity, have suggested that they may display positive cooperativity.[38] The findings detailed above may be histochemical and immunohistologic corroboration of these multiple sites and the positive cooperativity existing between them.

**B. Clinical Correlations with 17-FE and DCC**

At this point in time we have studied 150 cases of advanced breast cancer, assayed for EB with 17-FE, who were evaluable as to their response to endocrine manipulation. ER by DCC was available in 144. Twenty-eight of these patients were also in the group of women examined with 6-FE and ERICA.

Of the 150, 72 were positive for cytoplasmic EB. Forty-one (57%) responded to treatment or evidenced stabilization of disease. There were 48 17-FE-negative cases, of whom 44 (92%) failed. There were 30 patients whose tumors evidenced significant nuclear binding of 17-FE of whom 23 (77%) failed and 7 (23%) responded. The sensitivity of a positive, cytoplasmic 17-FE assay was 79% and the specificity 68% if nuclear EB is equated with a negative assay (Table 7).

There were 107 patients who were DCC+ (>3 fmol/mg protein). Forty-seven (44%) responded or were stabilized. There were 37 ER− cases of whom 34 (92%) failed. In this series, the sensitivity of DCC was 94% and the specificity 36% (Table 8).

If we assume that DCC identifies type I ER and 17-FE at least one subgroup of type II ER and that positive cooperativity exists between the two binding sites, then it would be

**Table 9**

**COMPARISON OF COMBINED ASSAY RESULTS
WITH 17-FE AND DCC AND CLINICAL
ENDOCRINE RESPONSE IN BREAST CANCER**

(Series 2)

| Assay results | Cases (#) | Failed (#) | Responded (#) | Stable (#) |
|---|---|---|---|---|
| 17-FE + /DCC + | 59 | 23 | 34 | 2 |
| 17-FE − /DCC − | 19 | 18 | 1 | 0 |
| 17-FE + /DCC − | 7 | 5 | 2 | 0 |
| 17-FE − /DCC + | 25 | 22 | 2 | 1 |
| 17-FE nuclear/DCC + | 23 | 14 | 9 | 0 |
| 17-FE nuclear/DCC − | 11 | 11 | 0 | 0 |

expected that the combined results of DCC and 17-FE would yield a better predictive value than either assay alone, and, indeed, this turns out to be the case (Table 9). Of the 144 cases where both ER and EB results were known, 59 were positive by both assays, of whom 36 (61%) either responded to hormonal therapy or became stabilized. There were 19 patients negative by both assays, 18 (95%) of whom failed. Twenty-three women were DCC + and showed nuclear EB. Nine (39%) responded while 14 (61%) failed. Eleven patients who were DCC − and exhibited nuclear EB also failed therapy. Of the remaining 32 women where either one or the other assay was negative (EB + ER −; EB − ER +), only 5 (16%) responded; the other 27 (84%) failed. The sensitivity of these combined assay systems was 71% and the specificity 75% provided that the patients showing nuclear 17-FE were considered as negative.

## C. Clinical Correlations with the Addition of Progesterone Binding Data

About 40% of women with ER + breast cancers fail hormonal therapy. It has been postulated that this might be due to postbinding defects in the pathway of estrogen activity. Since the synthesis of progesterone receptor (PgR) is apparently dependent upon proper functioning ER, then determination of PgR should improve the predictive value of biochemical steroid hormone assays[39] and, perhaps, also, of histochemical progesterone binding (PB) studies.

PgR was available on 96 of the 150 patients. PB by histochemistry had been determined on 145. The latter was performed utilizing 11 alpha-hydroxyprogesterone-bovine serum albumin-fluorescein isothiocyanate (11FP)[40] in a concentration of $7 \times 10^{-7}$ $M$, with the addition of a 100-fold excess molar concentration of hydrocortisone and dihydrotestosterone to inhibit binding to glucocorticoid and androgen receptors. The criteria for positivity was the same as for 17-FE, i.e., >10% positively stained tumor cells exhibiting at least a +1 cytoplasmic fluorescence intensity. Biochemical PgR positivity was assigned to specimens containing >5 fmol/mg protein.

Results of PgR and PB were available for correlation in 96 patients. There was concordance as to positivity and negativity in 70%. Ten patients with tumors which were PgR + were PB −, and 11 cases which were PgR − were PB + . Seventeen showed predominantly nuclear PB. Nine of the latter were PgR + and eight were PgR − (Table 10).

## D. ER and PgR by Biochemical Assay: Clinical Correlations

The addition of PgR data improved the predictive values of the biochemical steroid receptor assays (Table 11). There were 44 patients who were ER + PgR + of whom 26 (59%)

**Table 10**
**COMPARISON OF PgR BY**
**BIOCHEMISTRY AND**
**PROGESTERONE BINDING BY**
**HISTOCHEMISTRY**

(Series 2)

|         | PB + | PB − | PB-nuclear | Total |
|---------|------|------|------------|-------|
| PgR +   | 28   | 10   | 9          | 47    |
| PgR −   | 11   | 30   | 8          | 49    |
| Total   | 39   | 40   | 17         | 96    |

*Note:* PB = progesterone binding.

**Table 11**
**COMPARISON OF ER AND PgR ASSAY**
**RESULTS BY BIOCHEMISTRY WITH**
**CLINICAL ENDOCRINE RESPONSE IN**
**BREAST CANCER**

(Series 2)

| Assay results | Cases (#) | Failed (#) | Responded (#) | Stable (#) |
|---------------|-----------|------------|---------------|------------|
| ER + PgR +    | 44        | 18         | 24            | 2          |
| ER − PgR −    | 20        | 17         | 3             | 0          |
| ER + PgR −    | 29        | 23         | 6             | 0          |
| ER − PgR +    | 3         | 3          | 0             | 0          |
| Total         | 96        | 61         | 33            | 2          |

responded to hormonal manipulation or had their disease stabilized. Twenty women were ER − PgR − of whom 17 (85%) failed therapy. Twenty-nine patients were ER + PgR − . Six (21%) responded while 23 (79%) failed. Sensitivity was 74% and specificity 70%.

### E. EB and PB by Histochemistry: Clinical Correlations

Results of both EB and PB were available on 145 patients (Table 12). Forty-eight were EB + PB + of whom 29 (60%) responded. Forty-four were EB − PB − of which group 42 (96%) progressed. Two patients were EB − PB + . One responded while the other progressed. Fifteen were EB + PB − . Five (33%) responded and ten (67%) progressed. Eighteen patients exhibited nuclear EB and PB. Four responded while 14 failed. Three patients showed nuclear EB and were PB − and all failed. Six women displayed cytoplasmic EB and nuclear PB. Four (75%) responded and two progressed. Eight showed nuclear EB and cytoplasmic PB. Four responded and four failed. The remaining patient was EB − with nuclear PB and failed. The sensitivity of these combined histochemical assays was 59% with a specificity of 80%, considering nuclear binding to be equated with a negative assay.

### F. Combined ER, PgR, EB, and PB Assay Results: Clinical Correlations

Although to our knowledge type II PgR binding sites have not yet been described, it is reasonable to assume that low-affinity binding sites also exist for progesterone, may be of

**Table 12**

**COMPARISON OF COMBINED ESTROGEN AND PROGESTERONE BINDING RESULTS BY HISTOCHEMISTRY WITH CLINICAL ENDOCRINE RESPONSE IN BREAST CANCER**

(Series 2)

| Assay results | Cases (#) | Failed (#) | Responded (#) | Stable (#) |
|---|---|---|---|---|
| EB + PB + | 48 | 19 | 27 | 2 |
| EB − PB − | 44 | 42 | 1 | 1 |
| EB − PB + | 2 | 1 | 1 | 0 |
| EB + PB − | 15 | 10 | 5 | 0 |
| EB − nuclear/PB − nuclear | 18 | 14 | 4 | 0 |
| EB − nuclear/PB + | 8 | 4 | 4 | 0 |
| EB − nuclear/PB − | 3 | 3 | 0 | 0 |
| EB + PB − nuclear | 6 | 2 | 4 | 0 |
| EB − PB − nuclear | 1 | 1 | 0 | 0 |

*Note:* EB = estrogen binding with 17-FE, PB = progesterone binding.

**Table 13**

**COMPARISON OF COMBINED HISTOCHEMICAL ESTROGEN AND PROGESTERONE BINDING ASSAYS WITH CLINICAL ENDOCRINE RESPONSE IN BREAST CANCER**

(Series 2)

| Assay results | Cases (#) | Failed (#) | Responded (#) | Stable (#) |
|---|---|---|---|---|
| EB + PB + ER + PgR + | 23 | 6 | 16 | 1 |
| EB − /N PB − /N ER − PgR − | 9 | 9 | 0 | 0 |
| Any one assay negative (nuclear) | 14 | 7 | 7 | 0 |
| Any two assays negative (nuclear) | 28 | 19 | 8 | 1 |
| Any three assays negative (nuclear) | 19 | 19 | 0 | 0 |

*Note:* EB = estrogen binding, PB = progesterone binding by histochemistry, and N = nuclear ligand binding by histochemistry.

physiological importance, and may be identified by histochemistry. If this is the case, then the best overall predictive values should result when all the data are combined, providing that there is positive cooperativity between all sites. Our data suggest that this is, indeed, the case (Table 13).

Combined estrogen and progesterone biochemical and histochemical binding data were available in 93 cases. Twenty-three women were positive by all assay systems and 17 (74%) responded or became stable. Nine patients were either negative or showed nuclear binding in any one histochemical test. All of them failed therapy. Of interest, out of the remaining 61 cases, the percentage progressing was directly related to the number of negative (or nuclear) assays. Thus, if any one assay was negative (nuclear), 50% progressed on endocrine treatment. If any two assays were negative (nuclear), 68% progressed, while if three were negative/nuclear, 100% failed. Although combining the results of the assays increased the

**Table 14**
## COMPARISON OF PREDICTIVE VALUES, SENSITIVITIES, AND SPECIFICITIES OF HISTOCHEMICAL AND BIOCHEMICAL STEROID HORMONE BINDING ASSAYS, ALONE AND IN COMBINATION

| Type of assay | Cases (#) | Predictive value of positive assay (%) | Predictive value of negative assay (%) | Specificity (%) | Sensitivity (%) |
|---|---|---|---|---|---|
| Series 1 | | | | | |
| ERICA | 32 | 88 | 88 | 88 | 88 |
| DCC | 31 | 64 | 78 | 47 | 88 |
| 6-FE | 32 | 56 | 71 | 31 | 88 |
| 17-FE | 32 | 64 | 100 | 44 | 100 |
| Above combined | 31 | 100 | 80 | 100 | 75 |
| Series 2 | | | | | |
| DCC (ER) | 144 | 44 | 92 | 36 | 94 |
| DCC and 17-FE | 144 | 61 | 95 | 75 | 71 |
| 17-FE | 150 | 57 | 92 | 68 | 79 |
| ER and PgR | 96 | 59 | 85 | 70 | 74 |
| EB and PB | 145 | 60 | 96 | 79 | 59 |
| Above combined | 93 | 74 | 100 | 90 | 53 |

*Note:* EB = estrogen binding with 17-FE, PB = progesterone binding by histochemistry.

predictive value of positive assays and, thus, the specificity, there was some loss of sensitivity (Table 14).

### G. Other Histochemical-Clinical Correlations

At this time we are aware of two other studies in which results of histochemistry were correlated with clinical endocrine response of breast cancer. Yao et al.[41] studied a group of 28 women with 6-FE. All received cytotoxic chemotherapy. Ten were EB + of whom nine were additionally treated with hormonal therapy. Of the EB + patients, 89% responded. Six other patients who were EB − were also treated hormonally. Of the latter group, 83% progressed. In this series, the percentage of EB + responders is higher than in our own. However, the number of cases is small and the patients were all on multiple therapies. We have not as yet correlated our own data with response to multiple therapeutic modalities.

In the brief abstract of Sismondi et al.,[22] there is a statement that there was no evidence of correlation of ER and PgR via the Lee method with clinical outcome. However, there is no indication of the number of patients studied or of the results of the various assays and, therefore, this study cannot be evaluated at this time.

## V. DIFFERENCES BETWEEN 6-FE AND 17-FE

The reasons underlying the incongruities between the binding of 6-FE and 17-FE appear to be relatively complex. In the first place, these two conjugates are quite different in their molecular structure and, therefore, the stoichiometry of each is quite likely different. During the synthesis of 6-FE, estradiol is bound to BSA at position 6 whereas for 17-FE the 17 position is utilized. In 6-FE, a carboxymethyloxime bridge is employed, while for 17-FE the bridge is a hemisuccinate. 6-FE contains anywhere from 20 to 30 mol of estradiol derivative and up to 10 mol of fluorescein per mole BSA.[42] 17-FE contains 4 to 6 mol of both steroid and fluorescein. In addition, the techniques employed for each ligand-conjugate are somewhat different. For 6-FE, the tissue sections are first rehydrated and there is no postfixation step. For 17-FE, the sections are not rehydrated and the tissues are postfixed in ethanol-acetone. Also, for 17-FE, a 10% ethanol diluent is used in order to permit the addition of competitor ligands. Lastly, the concentration of 6-FE approaches $2 \times 10^{-4} M$ whereas for 17-FE the working concentration is $7 \times 10^{-7} M$.

The antiestrogen nafoxidine hydrochloride (CI-628), at 100-fold the molar concentration of 17-FE, results in a 90 to 100% inhibition of binding of 17-FE. Tamoxifen and diethylstilbestrol also inhibit the binding of 17-FE in somewhat higher concentrations. It is difficult to perform similar experiments with 6-FE since the concentrations of competitor required exceed the solubility limits of these agents.

In experiments designed to elucidate the nature of the binding patterns produced by 6-FE and 17-FE, we have found that concentration of conjugate is an important factor. When 6-FE is employed at a concentration of $7 \times 10^{-7} M$, little or no staining can be seen whether or not the tissue sections are postfixed. On the other hand, when 17-FE is used at concentrations approaching $2 \times 10^{-4} M$, the background staining becomes disconcertingly high. Furthermore, cytoplasmic staining becomes visible in tumor cells which only had exhibited nuclear staining at the lesser concentration. However, reducing the concentration of 6-FE does not result in nuclear staining but only in a reduction of cytoplasmic fluorescence.

Previously we have shown that breast cancer specimens demonstrating cytoplasmic binding with 17-FE often show nuclear fluorescence after incubation in tissue culture medium in the presence of estrogens at 37°C.[43] When exposed to 6-FE, however, the staining pattern remains cytoplasmic as it appeared in the nonincubated specimen.

That there are real and valid differences in the binding of 6-FE and 17-FE can also be demonstrated by microfluorometry (Figures 5A and B). Tissue sections which show only one peak with 17-FE, indicating one population of binding cells, not infrequently exhibit multiple peaks with 6-FE. The latter finding indicates the presence of several cell populations of varying binding capacity. Neither are the differences between 6-FE and 17-FE due to the technique employed. When 6-FE is employed as ligand in the Pertschuk method, the pattern produced is that of 6-FE when used in the Lee procedure, while using 17-FE in the Lee procedure, at a concentration of $7 \times 10^{-7} M$, produces the same imagery as when it is used in the Pertschuk technique.

These experiments clearly suggest that 6-FE and 17-FE intrinsically bind at different sites. Since one of the major differences does seem to be due to the concentration of ligand-conjugate which is used, it may be that 6-FE identifies so-called type III ER and that 17-FE binds to type II ER. Another possibility is that there exists at least two subgroups of type II ER, one recognized by 6-FE, the other by 17-FE. Be that as it may, our preliminary clinical data indicates that patients whose breast cancers are positive with both the fluorescent estrogens more often respond to endocrine therapy than patients whose tumors bind only one or the other conjugate, provided that type I ER is also present. This data also implies that there is positive cooperativity between these binding sites.

There are also factors which appear to indicate that 17-FE does not bind to type II ER. Clark and colleagues have shown that there is both a nuclear and cytoplasmic type II ER and that the cytoplasmic form is incapable of nuclear translocation. Additionally, nuclear type II ER estrogen binding is inhibited by dithiothreitol (DTT; 36,44,45). In our laboratory, the addition of up to 1 m/$M$ DTT does not inhibit nuclear binding of 17-FE.[5] Also, not only can nuclear binding and translocation be detected with 17-FE, when it is seen, there often appears to be little or no residual cytoplasmic fluorescence.[43] Nenci and co-workers[46] have made similar observations. This experimental work suggests that type I rather than type II ER is being identified.

Some time ago we reported that prostate tissue sections from specimens secured by electrocautery showed more nuclear binding by histochemistry than did specimens obtained via procedures which did not employ heat.[47] In experiments designed to investigate this phenomenon, thought to be related to heat-induced nuclear translocation, we studied parallel

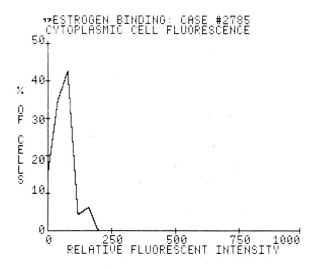

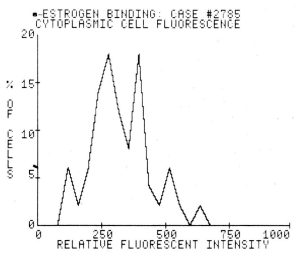

FIGURE 5. (A) Computer-derived graph of microfluorometer measurements of 17-FE bound by infiltrating duct cell carcinoma. One peak of cells showing relatively low ($\pm$) binding is evident. (B) Parallel section of same tumor reacted with 6-FE. The graph now shows five peaks indicative of five groups of cells with binding capacities varying from $\pm$ (125 units of relative fluorescent intensity) to $+3$ (750 units).

samples of breast cancer from six patients secured by electrocautery and by cold knife excision. All were then subjected to both 17-FE and biochemical assay for nuclear ER in a double-blind manner.[5] Five samples showed cytoplasmic fluorescence in the portion obtained without heat and nuclear staining in the portion secured by electrocautery. In all specimens, there was a significantly increased nuclear ER by biochemical assay in the latter tissue blocks. These studies which document measurable and visibly increased nuclear ER in the same tissue specimens are also more consistent with identification of type I rather than type II ER.

## VI. NUCLEAR BINDING OF 17-FE

In these studies we have shown that the presence of a large number of tumor cells with nuclear-bound 17-FE is an unfavorable prognostic sign in the prediction of response to endocrine therapies. We now have data indicating that nuclear 17-FE is also a marker of a more aggressive breast neoplasm.

In an analysis of crude survival time of the more than 750 patients currently enrolled in these studies, it was found that only 59% of patients with lesions displaying primarily nuclear 17-FE were alive at 2 years as compared with 78% of cases with principally cytoplasmic 17-FE. By 3 years, these figures were 49 vs. 69% survival (nuclear vs. cytoplasmic). A mixed pattern of nuclear and cytoplasmic 17-FE also was related to survival. Although not as apparent at 2 and 3 years, by 4 years only 46% of these cases were alive as compared to 66% of those with cytoplasmic 17-FE.

Nuclear 17-FE was an indicator of poor survival even in the presence of a positive ER by DCC (>10 fmol/mg protein). At 2 years, the survival of ER+ 17-FE-nuclear cases was 53% compared to 75% for ER+ 17-FE-cytoplasmic cases. At 4 years, the survival of ER+ 17-FE-mixed nuclear/cytoplasmic cases was 47% compared to 70% survival for ER+ 17-FE-cytoplasmic cases. Why nuclear 17-FE should be a poor prognostic indicator both of response to hormonal therapy as well as survival is not known at this time. Perhaps persisting nuclear 17-FE indicates a breakdown in the normal pathway of action of estradiol and this defect is more likely to occur in aggressive tumors.

In summary, the exact nature and significance of the binding sites revealed by histo-chemical assays remain unclear. What is now apparent is that there exists a multiplicity of estrogen and other steroid hormone binding sites in endocrine responsive cells and that histochemical and biochemical steroid binding assay systems can be used to complement each other. Close cooperation between investigators in both disciplines should eventually lead to a better understanding of the complex mechanism of action of steroids in target tissues. Possibilities that some of the discrepancies which appear to exist may be due to artifacts in biochemical[48] as well as in histochemical analytical methods should also be explored.

## ACKNOWLEDGMENTS

Ms. Evelyn Rainford and Ms. Ethel Jones supplied valued technical expertise. Dr. Eric Gaetjens supplied the estrogen (17-FE) and progesterone ligand-conjugates. Zeus Scientific, Inc., Raritan, N. J. generously donated 6-FE. We are grateful for the gifts of D547 Spγ and D75 Spγ monoclonal estrophilin antibodies provided by Dr. G. L. Greene. Warner-Lamber/Parke-Davis donated CI-628.

## REFERENCES

1. **DeSombre, E. R., Carbone, P. P., Jensen, E. V., McGuire, W. L., Wells, S. A., Jr., Wittliff, J. L., and Lipsett, M. B.,** Steroid receptors in breast cancer, *N. Engl. J. Med.*, 301, 1011, 1979.
2. **Chamness, G. C., Mercer, W. D., and McGuire, W. L.,** Are histochemical methods for estrogen receptor valid?, *J. Histochem. Cytochem.*, 28, 792, 1980.
3. **Chamness, G. C. and McGuire, W. L.,** Questions about histochemical methods for steroid receptors, *Arch. Pathol. Lab. Med.*, 106, 53, 1982.
4. **Stumpf, W. F.,** The histochemistry of steroid hormone "receptors", *J. Histochem. Cytochem.*, 31, 113, 1983.

5. **Pertschuk, L. P., Tobin, E. H., Carter, A. C., Eisenberg, K. B., Leo, V. C., Gaetjens, E., and Bloom, N. D.,** Immunohistologic and histochemical methods for detection of steroid binding in breast cancer: a reappraisal, *Breast Cancer Res. Treat.,* 1, 297, 1981.
6. **Greene, G. L., Fitch, F. W., and Jensen, E. V.,** Monoclonal antibodies to estrophilin: probes for the study of estrogen receptors, *Proc. Natl. Acad. Sci. U.S.A.,* 77, 157, 1980.
7. **Greene, G. L., Nolan, C., Engler, J. P., and Jensen, E. V.,** Monoclonal antibodies to human estrogen receptor, *Proc. Natl. Acad. Sci. U.S.A.,* 77, 5115, 1981.
8. **King, W. J. and Greene, G. L.,** Monoclonal antibodies localize oestrogen receptor in the nuclei of target cells, *Nature (London),* 307, 745, 1984.
9. **Press, M. F., King, W., and Greene, G.,** Immunocytochemical localization of estrogen receptors in the human endometrium using a monoclonal antibody against human estrogen receptor, *Fed. Proc.,* 42, 1178, 1983.
10. **Lee, S. H.,** Hydrophilic macromolecules of steroid derivatives for the detection of cancer cell receptors, *Cancer,* 46, 2825, 1980.
11. **Pertschuk, L. P., Gaetjens, E., Carter, A. C., Brigati, D. J., Kim, D. S., and Fealey, T. E.,** An improved histochemical method for detection of estrogen receptors in mammary cancer, *Am. J. Clin. Pathol.,* 71, 504, 1979.
12. **Hasson, J.,** Disappointing results, *Am. J. Clin. Pathol.,* 77, 377, 1982.
13. **Bohm, M. P., Binder, M., and Czenwenka, K.,** Evaluation of biochemical and staining properties of direct and indirect immunohistochemical methods for detection of steroid binding proteins, presented at the 11th Int. Conf. Clin. Chem., Vienna, August 31, 1981.
14. **Jacobs, S. R., Wolfson, W. L., Cheng, L., and Lewin, K. J.,** Cytochemical and competitive protein binding assays for estrogen receptor in breast disease, *Cancer,* 51, 1621, 1983.
15. **Alonso, K. and Brownlee, N.,** Estrogen receptors by immunofluorescence: comparison with a dextran-coated charcoal assay, *Ann. Clin. Lab. Sci.,* 11, 132, 1981.
16. **Tominaga, T., Kitamura, M., Saito, T., Itoh, I., and Takikawa, H.,** Comparative histochemical and biochemical assay of estrogen receptors in breast cancer patients, *Gann,* 72, 60, 1981.
17. **Hanna, W., Ryder, R. E., and Mobbs, B. G.,** Cellular localization of estrogen binding in human breast cancer, *Am. J. Clin. Pathol.,* 77, 391, 1982.
18. **Meijer, C. J. L. M., van Marle, J., Persijn, J. P., van Niewenhuizen, W., Baak, J. P. A., Boon, M. E., and Lindeman, J.,** Estrogen receptors in human breast cancer. II. Correlation between the histochemical method and biochemical assay, *Virchows Arch. (Cell Pathol.),* 40, 27, 1982.
19. **Berger, G., Frapport, L., Berger, N., Bremond, A., Ferold, J., and Rochet, Y.,** Localisation cytoplasmique des recepteurs steroidiens des carcinomes mammaires par histofluorescence, *Arch. Anat. Cytol. Pathol.,* 28, 341, 1980.
20. **O'Connell, M. D. and Said, J. W.,** Estrogen receptors in carcinoma of the breast. A comparison of the dextran-coated charcoal, immunofluorescent and immunoperoxidase technics, *Am. J. Clin. Pathol.,* 80, 1, 1983.
21. **Panko, W. B., Mattioli, C. A., and Wheeler, T. M.,** Lack of correlation of a histochemical method for estrogen receptor analysis with the biochemical assay results, *Cancer,* 49, 2148, 1982.
22. **Sismondi, P., Barengo, R., Botta, R., De Tetto, F., Giardina, G., Mano, M. P., Preve, C. U., Sussio, M., Zola, P., and Bocci, A.,** Prognostic values of estrogen receptors (ER) and progesterone receptors (PgR) as determined by radiochemical and histochemical methods in breast cancer — a multicentric experience, *Breast Cancer Res. Treat.,* 2, 279, 1982.
23. **Davis, J. R., Penney, R. J., and Graham, A. R.,** personal communication, 1981.
24. **Stumpf, W. E. and Roth, L. J.,** High resolution autoradiography with dry-mounted, freeze-dried, frozen sections. Comparative study of six methods using two different compounds ($^3$H)-estradiol and ($^3$H)-meso-bilirubinogen, *J. Histochem. Cytochem.,* 14, 274, 1966.
25. **Stumpf, W. E. and Sar, M.,** Autoradiographic localization of estrogen, androgen, progestin and glucocorticosteroid in "target tissues" and "non-target tissues", in *Receptors and Mechanism of Action of Steroid Hormones, Modern Pharmacology-Toxicology,* Vol. 8, Pasquilini, J., Ed., Marcel Dekker, New York, 1976, 41.
26. **Buell, R. H. and Tremblay, G.,** The localization of $^3$H-estradiol in estrogen receptor-positive human mammary carcinoma as visualized by thaw-mount autoradiography, *Cancer,* 51, 1625, 1983.
27. **Sheridan, P. J.,** Is there an alternative to the cytoplasmic receptor model for the mechanism of action of steroids?, *Life Sci.,* 17, 497, 1975.
28. **Martin, P. M. and Sheridan, P. J.,** Intracellular distribution of estrogen receptors; a function of preparation, *Experientia,* 36, 620, 1980.

29. **Pertschuk, L. P., Eisenberg, K. B., Leo, V. C., Rainford, E. A., Carter, A. C., and Macchia, R. J.,** Immunofluorescence detection of estrogen receptors with monoclonal antibodies. Clinical correlation of steroid binding by histochemistry in breast and prostate carcinoma, in *Proc. 11th Int. Congr. Clin. Chem.,* Kaiser, E., Gabl, F., Mueller, M. M., and Bayer, M., Eds., Walter de Gruyter, Berlin, 1982, 493.

30. **Nadji, M. and Morales, A. R.,** Immunocytochemistry of estrogen receptors in breast cancer, presented at the 7th Int. Conf. on Defined Immunofluorescence, Immunoenzyme Studies and Related Labeling Techniques, Niagara Falls, N.Y., June 2, 1982.

31. **Garancis, J. C., Miller, L. S., Tomita, J. T., Tieu, T. M., and Clowry, L. J., Jr.,** Immunoperoxidase localization of estrogen receptors in human breast carcinoma, *Cancer Detection Prev.,* 6, 235, 1983.

32. **Raam, S., Nemeth, I. J., Tamura, H., O'Briain, D. S., and Cohen, J. L.,** Immunohistochemical localization of estrogen receptors in human mammary carcinoma using antibodies to the receptor protein, *Eur. J. Cancer Clin. Oncol.,* 18, 1, 1982.

33. **Raam, S., Richardson, G. S., Bradley, F., MacLaughlin, D., Sun, L., Frankel, F., and Cohen, J. L.,** Translocation of cytoplasmic estrogen receptors to the nucleus: immunohistochemical demonstration utilizing rabbit antibodies to estrogen receptors of mammary carcinomas, *Breast Cancer Res. Treat.,* 3, 179, 1983.

34. **Mercer, W. D., Lippman, M. E., Wahl, T. M., Carlson, C. A., Wahl, D. A., Lezotte, D., and Teague, P. O.,** The use of immunocytochemical techniques for the detection of steroid hormones in breast cancer cells, *Cancer,* 46, 2859, 1980.

35. **Clark, J. H. and Peck, E. J., Jr., Eds.,** *Female Sex Steroids. Receptors and Function,* Springer-Verlag, Berlin, 1979.

36. **Markaverich, B. M., Williams, M., Upchurch, S., and Clark, J. H.,** Heterogeneity of nuclear estrogen-binding sites in the rat uterus: a simple method for the quantitation of type I and type II sites by ($^3$H) estradiol exchange, *Endocrinology,* 109, 62, 1981.

37. **Panko, W. B., Watson, C. S., and Clark, J. H.,** The presence of a second, specific estrogen binding site in human breast cancer, *J. Steroid Biochem.,* 14, 1311, 1981.

38. **Clark, J. H., Watson, C. S., Markaverich, B. M., Syne, J. S., and Panko, W. B.,** Heterogeneity of estrogen binding sites in mammary tumors, *Breast Cancer Res. Treat.,* 3, 61, 1983.

39. **Horwitz, K. B., McGuire, W. L., Pearson, O. H., and Segaloff, A.,** Predicting response to endocrine therapy in human breast cancer: an hypothesis, *Science,* 189, 726, 1975.

40. **Pertschuk, L. P., Tobin, E. H., Gaetjens, E., Degenshein, G. A., Autuoro, L. M., Brigati, D. J., Bloom, N. D., Carter, A. C., and Rainford, E. A.,** A histochemical technique for evaluation of progesterone receptors in breast cancer, *Res. Commun. Chem. Pathol. Pharmacol.,* 23, 635, 1979.

41. **Yao, X., Meng, X., Chen, P., and Mei, Z.,** Histochemical estrogen receptor assay for selecting stage III breast cancers for combined chemohormonal therapy, *Lab. Invest.,* 48, 96A, 1983.

42. **Lee, S. H.,** Cytochemical study of estrogen receptor in human mammary carcinoma, *Am. J. Clin. Pathol.,* 70, 197, 1978.

43. **Pertschuk, L. P., Gaetjens, E., Carter, A. C., and Macchia, R. J.,** Histochemical detection of estrogen receptor translocation in breast and prostate tumors, *Fed. Proc.,* 39, 414, 1980.

44. **Eriksson, H., Upchurch, S., Hardin, J. W., Peck, E. J., Jr., and Clark, J. H.,** Heterogeneity of estrogen receptors in the cytosol and nuclear fractions of the rat uterus, *Biochem. Biophys. Res. Commun.,* 81, 1, 1978.

45. **Markaverich, B. M. and Clark, J. H.,** Two binding sites for estradiol in rat uterine nuclei; relationship to uterotropic response, *Endocrinology,* 105, 1458, 1979.

46. **Nenci, I., Fabris, G., Mazzola, A., Bagni, A., Poli, G., and Marchetti, E.,** personal communication, 1983.

47. **Pertschuk, L. P., Rosenthal, H. E., Macchia, R. J., Eisenberg, K. B., Feldman, J. G., Wax, S. H., Kim, D. S., Whitmore, W. F., Jr., Abrahams, J. I., Gaetjens, E., Wise, G. J., Herr, H. W., Karr, J. P., Murphy, G. P., and Sandberg, A. A.,** Correlation of histochemical and biochemical analyses of androgen binding in prostatic cancer: relation to therapeutic response, *Cancer,* 49, 984, 1982.

48. **Melzer, M. S.,** Intracellular receptors for androgens: experimental artifact?, *Urology,* 21, 332, 1983.

Chapter 3

# A FLUORESCENT HISTOCHEMICAL STUDY OF STEROID RECEPTORS IN HUMAN BREAST CANCER

**Sin Hang Lee**

## TABLE OF CONTENTS

I.      Introduction .................................................................. 38

II.     Historical Background ...................................................... 39

III.    Specificity of the Technique for ER Assay ............................ 39

IV.     Applications in Diagnostic Pathology .................................. 43
        A.      Infiltrating Mammary Carcinomas ........................... 43
        B.      Malignant Effusions .......................................... 45
        C.      Biology of Potentially Hormone-Responsive Cancers ..... 46
        D.      Applications in Other Cancers ............................... 47

V.      Concluding Remarks ....................................................... 47

Acknowledgments ................................................................. 48

References ........................................................................ 48

## I. INTRODUCTION

For more than 10 years, the most extensively used approach to identify potentially hormone-responsive breast cancers is to measure soluble estrogen receptor (ER) proteins in the supernatant, the so-called cytosol fraction of the tumor tissue homogenates, using a dextran-coated charcoal (DCC) or a sucrose density gradient technique.[1,2] The quantity of ER proteins in the cytosol is usually expressed as estrogen binding capacity in femtomoles per gram of wet tissue or per milligram of proteins in solution. The rate of response to hormonal treatment, usually at about 30 to 60% for the ER-positive tumors, appears to be in proportion to the estrogen binding capacity of the tumor proteins.[3,4]

The urgent need for a practical histochemical technique which can be used to distinguish between ER-negative and ER-positive cancers was quickly recognized by the pathologists[5-7] as soon as the technology of the ER protein assays extended beyond the boundaries of the few large, federally funded biochemical laboratories. It is the professional instinct that drives the pathologists to venture out of their traditional morphological domain to search for an alternative approach to evaluate ER status of a tumor. The reason is very simple, for no one knows better than the pathologist how heterogeneous in cellular composition the specimens of human breast cancer really are. Should there be a common denominator in these specimens, a denominator that can be used to denote a function of the malignant cells, it certainly will not be the wet weight of the specimen or the extractable proteins thereof, because in breast cancer the malignant cells are often scattered as islands or singly between benign mammary ducts or admixed with inflammatory cells, making an exclusive extraction of any cancerous components almost impossible. The ER level obtained with biochemical assays, in fact, represents no more than estrogen binding capacity of a mixed pool of proteins derived not only from the cancer cells, but also from the benign epithelial cells, the myoepithelial cells, the stromal cells, the inflammatory cells, the plasma, and the interstitial fluid. How accurately this numerical level reflects the physiological status of the cancer cell population in the specimen naturally to a large extent depends on the histological composition of the tumor mass submitted for assay.

A histochemical technique, on the other hand, can provide a means to evaluate a function of a specific cell type, for example, the infiltrating cancer cells, using the number of cancer cells under observation as the common denominator. Such an approach has also been used to study the intracellular estrogen receptors of the luminal epithelial cells of the rat uterus under different physiological and experimental conditions.[9-13]

From a practical standpoint, an ideal histochemical test, in the first place, should be able to predict the tumor response or the clinical course with a high accuracy, and second, should allow the results to be reproduced by independent workers in different laboratories with ease. Since 1978, a technique based on the use of a macromolecular hydrophilic fluorescent estradiol conjugate as a histochemical reagent for localizing the cells with a high estrogen binding capacity, or estrogen receptors, in cryostat sections has been made available to the practicing pathologists in many countries. During this short period of time, many preliminary reports have appeared in the literature and confirmed that the initial observation with this technique is reproducible,[14-23] that when the technique is used under optimum conditions and in experienced hands the histochemical assays are in 75 to 92% of the cases in agreement with the tumor ER protein values obtained with cytosolic analysis, and that the biological behaviors of the ER-rich and the ER-poor breast cancers identified by this histochemical test are similar to those of ER-rich and ER-poor tumors identified by the biochemical assays. In this chapter, the general principle of the methodology and several important aspects pertinent to the application of this technique in the practice of diagnostic pathology are discussed. The technical procedure has been the subject of a previous review[24] and, consequently, will not be covered in detail here.

## II. HISTORICAL BACKGROUND

After several attempts were made to use an indirect immunofluorescence approach to trace the in vitro binding of 17β-estradiol[5] and polyestradiol phosphate[6] in frozen sections, it was realized these multiple-step procedures can only yield reproducible results with great difficulties for various reasons.[24] Then, our effort was directed to the synthesis of a fluorescent estradiol hormone so that the steps requiring the use of high-titered antibodies can be obviated. The use of a hydrophilic molecule, such as the bovine serum albumin (BSA), as a carrier is deemed essential to maintain a high solubility of the steroid hormones in an aqueous solution at physiologic pH. It soon became clear that a BSA molecule carrying about 26 radicals of 17β-estradiol-6-carboxymethyl oxime and about 4 radicals of fluorescein iso-thiocyanate (FITC) covalently coupled to the carrier via carboxamide linkages proves to be a satisfactory reagent to stain the estrogen target cells in cryostat frozen sections of various tissues.[7,8,25]

The initial factual observations can be summarized as follows: a solution of BSA-FITC without the coupled estradiol derivative did not produce a differential staining in any tissue cryostat sections, cancerous or noncancerous. The fluorescent histochemical reagent must carry at least 20 mol of 17β-estradiol-6-carboxymethyl oxime per 1 mol of BSA to cause the cytoplasm of certain breast cancer cells in cryostat frozen sections to fluoresce intensely. With this technique, the infiltrating human breast carcinomas were found to be composed of highly heterogeneous cancer cells in terms of estrogen binding capacity which might be arbitrarily graded from negative ($-$) to strongly positive ($4+$). Only in about one third or less of the breast cancers surveyed, the number of cancer cells showing strongly cytoplasmic fluorescence equaled or exceeded the number of negative or weakly fluorescent cancer cells in the same tumor. Although breast cancers consisting of all ER-negative cancer cells were commonly encountered, constituting up to 20% of the randomly selected tumors, every breast cancer seemed to contain at least a few islands of nonfluorescent tumor cells. Like the cancer cells, the benign epithelial cells of the mammary ducts and lobules also showed varying degrees of cytoplasmic fluorescence; but the intensity of fluorescence in the benign epithelial cells usually did not reach that exhibited by the strongly positive breast cancer cells. The reproducibility of this histochemical technique was confirmed by staining several consecutive serial cryostat sections of the same tumor tissue block, and examining the pattern of distribution of the fluorescent cancer cells in each section. The results indicated that the histochemical reagent identified a functional characteristic shared by the tumor cells in islands or in clones; thus, the staining was not due to a haphazard deposition of reagent in the sections. Fixation of the cryostat frozen sections in 4% formaldehyde or by flame heating abolished the staining of the cancer cells completely. Immersing the cryostat frozen sections in cold acetone reduced the intensity of fluorescence depending on the duration of fixation. The cytoplasm of the smooth muscle cells of the human myometrium were often positive for the staining. But the smooth muscle cells of the bowel wall and blood vessels, and the cells in the lymph nodes, tonsils, spleen, and lungs were consistently negative. The epithelial cells and the stromal cells of the human endometrium were variable in staining. On the basis of these preliminary findings, it was concluded that the staining of the cells by this fluorescent reagent was most likely due to binding of the estradiol radicals by a relatively labile substance(s) in the cytoplasm of the estrogen target cells, probably a form of estrogen receptors.

## III. SPECIFICITY OF THE TECHNIQUE FOR ER ASSAY

The competitive radioactive isotope binding assays were originally developed in basic research laboratories to study the ER proteins in the homogenate of the uterus of the rodents.[26-28] Consequently, the uterus of the rat has become the model organ that is used for the study of female steroid hormone actions, including the methodology for receptor assays. On the other hand, the fluorescent histochemical technique was designed in a clinical laboratory for localization of cancer cell estrogen receptors of human carcinoma from the start. In order to prove that the histochemical technique is valid and capable of identifying the cells rich in estrogen receptors, it would be necessary to put this newly developed technique to test according to a set of proven criteria, or to measure it against a standardized method.

Numerous attempts have been made to correlate the histochemical findings with the cytosol ER assays on human breast cancer specimens. While many workers have reported a positive correlation between these two sets of data,[15-21,23] a few found the results disappointing.[29,30] There are at least three possible causes for a lack of correlations: (1) the biochemical techniques may not be as easily mastered as they are believed to be; (2) these two methods are designed to measure receptors of different cellular origins and, therefore, the results have no common denominator for a quantitative comparison; and (3) the estrogen binding sites revealed by the histochemical technique do not represent receptors.

First of all, although the dextran-coated charcoal and the sucrose density gradient techniques have been repeatedly declared "standardized" by individuals,[31] by an editorial of a medical journal,[32] and by a committee appointed by a U.S. federal agency,[33] the facts remain that aliquots of the same specimen of human breast cancer submitted to different laboratories for assay using these techniques are often reported to contain various levels of ER proteins, sometimes with a several-fold difference.[34,35] Only in laboratories with strict quality control measures can the results be reproducible. An entire international conference has been devoted to discuss the technical problems involved and the reports have been summarized in a monograph.[36] One example to further illustrate this point is the difficulty of using the cytosol assay to quantitate ER proteins of the rat uterus by different laboratories. It is well known that there is a regular cyclic fluctuation in the concentration of ER proteins in the uterus of the adult female rats during the estrous cycle. However, attempts to pinpoint the stage in which the concentration of the uterine ER proteins reaches its peak level have produced only contradicting results; it has been reported to occur at proestrus,[37] estrus,[38] and diestrus[39] by three different groups of researchers. Therefore, the lack of a biochemical assay which can be easily used by all laboratories to yield reproducible results has probably contributed to some of the failures in obtaining parallel correlations between the biochemical and the histochemical data.

Secondly, the heterogeneous nature of the human breast cancer specimen may have ruled out any possibility of obtaining an absolute parallel correlation between these two sets of data. The result of a histochemical assay is expressed in terms of percentage of ER-positive cells in an infiltrating cancer cell population, whereas the estrogen binding capacity per milligram of soluble proteins is used to report the cytosol assay. When a cancer specimen being studied is composed almost exclusively of malignant epithelial cells (Figure 1), the correlation between the histochemical and the biochemical data may be good. However, when a tumor contains very few scattered cancer cells (Figure 2), the correlation may be very poor because the biochemical assay measures largely the function of extractable proteins from the noncancerous cells to which the examiner of a histochemical preparation may pay little attention.

Finally, a histochemical technique should be verified on its own merits. The crucial question to ask is whether the estrogen binding activity localized by this fluorescent histochemical reagent is a function of true estrogen receptors. According to the established definition, a steroid receptor must bind its ligand with a high affinity, a limited capacity, hormone specificity, and tissue specificity, and must be correlated with biochemical response to the hormone action.[40] Experiments with cryostat frozen sections of the rat uterus have yielded convincing evidence that the cytoplasmic binding substance demonstrated by this technique, indeed, fulfills all of the criteria for the definition of estrogen receptors.[9-13] The

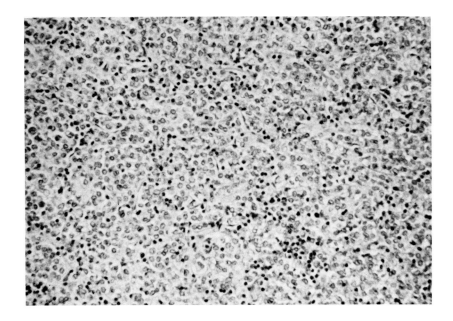

FIGURE 1. Photomicrograph of a metastatic lobular carcinoma in an axillary lymph node. Almost the entire specimen is composed of cancer cells. (H & E; magnification × 300.)

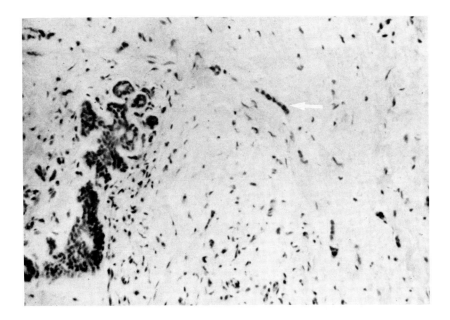

FIGURE 2. Infiltrating lobular carcinoma of the breast. This part of the specimen contains only a few cancer cells (arrows). Most of the epithelial cells shown in this photomicrograph are benign. (H & E; magnification × 300.)

cytoplasmic estrogen receptors in the luminal epithelial cells of the rat uterus prove to be most sensitive to the action of estrogens and antiestrogens, including tamoxifen.[13] A fluorescent histochemical technique seems to be most effective in identifying the cells with high concentrations of cytoplasmic receptors, such as the ER-rich epithelial cells of the uterus of the rat. An entire chapter in Volume 1 of this series has been devoted to this subject. Consequently, no attempt will be made to review this here.

The critics of this technique are usually those who are not familiar with the principles and the limitations of the histochemical methodology, in general. One group of authors criticized the use of unfixed cryostat frozen sections for ER assay, because in a biochemists' concept all receptor proteins would have leaked out of the cell once the cell membrane is ruptured or has been made permeable.[29] However, incubation of frozen sections of target tissues in media containing [³H]-estradiol proves that there is a large number of specific receptor sites retained in the tissue sections.[9,10,41] The binding sites are probably firmly attached to the cytoskeleton of the target cells. It is possible that only a small fraction of the estrogen receptors in the cells can be readily solubilized. Nevertheless, an inappropriate treatment of the specimens may well facilitate a breakdown of the cytoskeleton, causing uncontrollable dissociation of the cellular estrogen receptors from the tissue. For example, to store the specimens in a $-70°C$ refrigerator for different periods of time before processing them for histochemical staining, as reported by two groups,[29,30] may have accounted for their poor results in correlation with the biochemical assays and the clinical response rate of breast cancers. The best results are obtained if the specimens are processed for histochemical assay at a time when diagnostic frozen sections are made.

Another group objected to the use of histochemical staining solutions containing substances or ligands at a concentration much higher than the dissociation constant ($K_d$) of estrogen receptor proteins, claiming that at such high concentrations the ligand may stain many nonspecific binding proteins, such as the so-called type III binding sites — a loosely defined group of low-affinity estrogen binding proteins present in the tissue homogenate, including those of blood origin.[31] However, the critics have chosen to ignore an important fact that practically all histochemical procedures include a poststaining washing step. As the sections which have been stained are washed in a ligand-free solution, an equilibrium between the bound ligand and the free ligand will be eventually established in a system with a very low concentration of free ligand in solution. At the end of the washing step, it can be assumed that only the high-affinity binding sites would retain any significant amount of ligand for visualization. Although it is not known whether estrogen receptors in tissue sections can be subclassified into type I and type II sites like the proteins in cytosols of the rat uterus, the natural estrogens have been shown to dissociate rapidly from the type II binding proteins that have a much lower affinity for estradiol than the type I binders.[42,43] In fact, forcing the receptor proteins that have been initially oversaturated with ligand to migrate through a column of ligand-free solution to let the loosely bound ligand dissociate from the low-affinity binding sites is the principle used for distinguishing the type I and the type II receptors by the sucrose density gradient analysis. It seems reasonable to permit the same principle to be used in the histochemical assay to differentiate the low-affinity binding sites from the high-affinity binders. Whether all of the high-affinity estrogen binding sites localized in the cytoplasm would be capable of translocating into the nucleus in vivo is not clear.

There are fundamental differences in physicochemical characteristics between the soluble ER proteins being measured in a biochemical setting and the estrogen receptors in cryostat tissue sections. Unlike those soluble in dilute cytosols, the estrogen binding sites in the cytoplasm of an ER-rich breast cancer cell are not only bound to the cytoskeleton, but probably several hundred times more concentrated. It has been demonstrated that the binding sites in cryostat sections take a longer period of incubation to saturate, and like the immobilized enzymes, are probably governed by a special set of kinetic parameters.[44] It is entirely conceivable that it may require a rather high concentration of fluorescent ligand to give an adequate percentage of initial receptor saturation.

## IV. APPLICATIONS IN DIAGNOSTIC PATHOLOGY

### A. Infiltrating Mammary Carcinomas

One important application of the histochemical technique is to use it as a means to identify potentially hormone-responsive breast cancers. Such a technique may be employed as a supplementary to the cytosol assay or as an alternative, especially when the material is considered to be inadequate (Plate 1*) or not suitable for preparation of cytosols (Plates 2 and 3), and when the test is needed in the locations where no facilities for biochemical assays are available.

Since human breast cancers,[8] including the steroid-sensitive MCF-7 tumor cells in culture,[45] are so heterogeneous in cellular composition in terms of estrogen binding activity within the cancer cell population, it seems essential to define a cut-off line of cellular receptor positivity for correlating the histochemical assay results with other parameters. By comparative studies with the luminal epithelial cells of the rat uterus, and with the known hormone-sensitive and -insensitive cancer cells in culture, it is felt that the benign ductal epithelial cells of the human mammary gland that exhibit the highest intensity of cytoplasmic fluorescence are probably also highly sensitive to the change of hormonal milieu in vivo and, thus, could be chosen as an example of ER-positive epithelial cells; the cancer cells in the human breast tumor showing a similar degree of cytoplasmic fluorescence may be considered potentially sensitive to hormonal manipulation clinically and, therefore, labeled ER-positive. In addition, because a minimum 50% reduction in size of the entire known tumor mass has been accepted as a sign of regression according to the objective criteria for evaluating the effects of hormonal therapy, it has been suggested that a breast cancer containing a 50% or a higher proportion of ER-positive cells in the infiltrating cancer cell population be regarded as potentially hormone responsive.[46] Whether this proposed formula is the most suitable one would have to await publication of the works now in progress in many parts of the world. In his own experience, this author has not encountered a patient showing objective response to hormonal therapy when the breast cancer is composed of more than 95% ER-negative tumor cells. However, two cases of breast cancer that contain as low as 20% ER-positive cells in the cancer cell population have been known to respond to hormonal therapy alone. Perhaps, what eventually proves important may not be the level of a biological marker, such as the estrogen receptors, in the entire cancer cell population, but in those most aggressively growing tumor cells. It is not unusual to observe microscopically that within an island of infiltrating cancer cells the ER-positive ones are often located at the periphery. Experience with cell cultures has also indicated that the ER level of the actively growing MCF-7 tumor cells in early log phase is always higher than that in older cell cultures.[45] Nevertheless, most of the hormone-responsive breast cancers (Figures 3 and 4) have been those containing at least about 50% ER-positive cancer cells in the infiltrating cancer cell population.

In our laboratory, a combined histochemical reagent containing a mixture of 17β-estradiol-6-carboxymethyl oxime-BSA-FITC and 11α-hydroxyprogesterone hemisuccinate-BSA-tetramethylrhodamine isothiocyanate is routinely used.[47] All human breast cancer cells, benign human mammary ductal epithelial cells, and the luminal epithelial cells of the rat uterus that are positive for estrogen receptors have also been found to bind the progesterone reagent as well. This finding suggests that the cytoplasmic estrogen receptor and progesterone receptor in these epithelial cells probably appear either simultaneously or one following the other

---

* Plates 1 through 18 will appear following page 44.

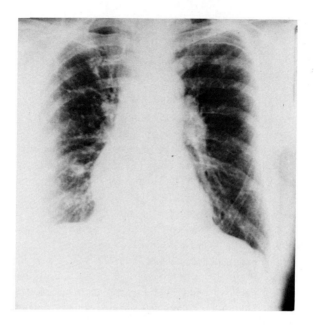

FIGURE 3.

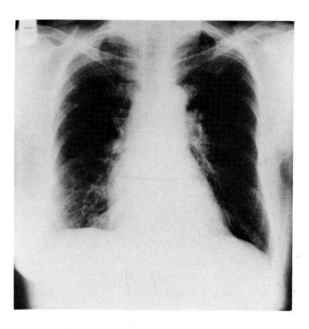

FIGURE 4.

FIGURE 3 and 4.    Case S80-9094. A 69-year-old female patient developed hilar lymph node enlargement and multiple densities on chest X-ray (Figure 3) 6 years after left radical mastectomy for a primary mammary carcinoma. All regional lymph nodes had been found to be negative at the time of mastectomy. Now the question of a possible second pulmonary primary arose. A 0.5 × 0.4 × 0.2 cm-tumor biopsy obtained through mediastinoscopy was submitted for a pathological diagnosis and steroid receptor assay. A poorly differentiated carcinoma in which over 90% of the cancer cells were positive for estrogen and progesterone receptors was confirmed by frozen sections. The patient was treated with tamoxifen only. Most of the pulmonary densities disappeared in 4 months (Figure 4).

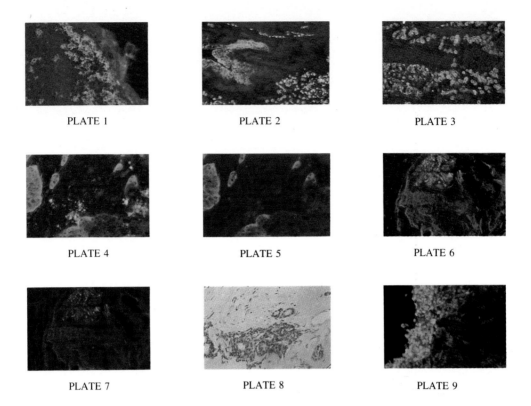

PLATE 1
PLATE 2
PLATE 3
PLATE 4
PLATE 5
PLATE 6
PLATE 7
PLATE 8
PLATE 9

PLATE 1.   A microscopic focus of metastatic mammary carcinoma in an axillary lymph node. The cancer cells showing apple-green fluorescence are positive for cytoplasmic estrogen receptors and are primarily located in the peripheral sinusoids. Cytosol assays invariably failed to detect the ER proteins in these specimens. (Magnification × 83.)

PLATES 2 and 3.   Case S81-6096. A primary mammary carcinoma (Plate 2) and its metastatic lesion in the wall of the stomach (Plate 3) showing largely ER-positive cancer cells in both specimens. These tumors were taken from a 47-year-old female patient who presented with gastric outlet obstruction and a mass in the left breast. Surgical exploration proved the stomach, the omentum, and the left breast were involved by poorly differentiated carcinomas. The gross and the microscopic appearance of the gastric lesion suggested a primary carcinoma of the stomach, linitis plastica. A histochemical assay showed that about 50% of the cancer cells in the breast tumor were positive for cytoplasmic estrogen and progesterone receptors. The tumor in the wall of the stomach was composed of 95% estrogen and progesterone receptor-positive cancer cells which were dispersed between bundles of smooth muscle cells. Tumor cytosol DCC assays by an independent regional laboratory reported 41 fmol of estrogen receptors and 18 fmol of progesterone receptors per milligram of proteins extracted from the breast tumor, and no receptors in the gastric cancer. Based on the results of the histochemical assay, the tumor was treated as a mammary carcinoma with metastases to the abdomen and proved to be hormone responsive during the course of $2^{1}/_{2}$ years clinical follow-up. This case illustrates the difficulty of measuring ER proteins of cancer cells in fibrous tissue and in smooth muscles. (Magnification × 83.)

PLATES 4 and 5.   A frozen section of a focally necrotic ductal carcinoma of the breast stained with a mixture of fluorescent estrogen and progesterone conjugates. The well-preserved ER-positive (apple-green) breast cancer cells also show progesterone binding activity (orange-red). Droplets of breakdown products derived from necrotic cancer cells bind only the estrogen reagent (Plate 4), but not the progesterone reagent (Plate 5). (Magnification × 83.)

PLATES 6, 7, and 8.   Two serial frozen sections showing foci of ER-negative mammary cancer cells infiltrating the stroma near a peripheral nerve. One section was stained with a mixed fluorescent estrogen and progesterone reagent (Plates 6 and 7), and the other with H & E (Plate 8). Note the binding of both the estrogen and progesterone compounds by the peripheral nerve, probably due to its high content of myelin. (Magnification × 83.)

PLATE 9.   An ER-negative mammary carcinoma with mechanically damaged cancer cells at the margin of the specimen, showing nonspecific fluorescence, apparently resulting from crush artifacts. (Magnification × 83.)

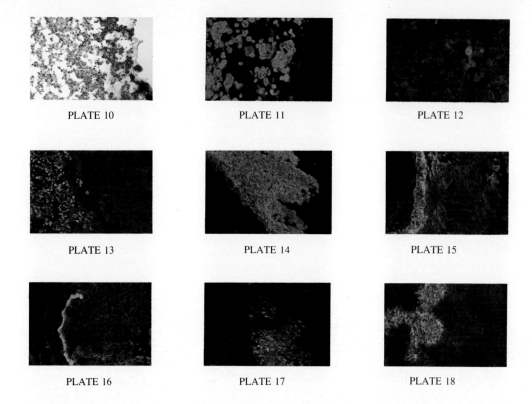

PLATE 10              PLATE 11              PLATE 12

PLATE 13              PLATE 14              PLATE 15

PLATE 16              PLATE 17              PLATE 18

PLATE 10 and 11.   Two serial cryostat frozen sections of a cell pellet derived from a pleural fluid specimen containing breast cancer cells, one stained for histochemical assay and the other with H & E. The cancer cells that are mixed with various numbers of mesothelial cells are usually settled above the layer of lymphocytes. (Plate 10, magnification × 52.) In this case, about 90% of the cancer cells are positive for estrogen and progesterone receptors. No cellular estrogen binding activity is noted in the lymphocytic band. (Plate 11, magnification × 83.)

PLATE 12.   Frozen section of a cell pellet consisting of cancer cells of a pleural effusion. After being stained in the histochemical reagent, all cancer cells were found to be negative for estrogen and progesterone receptors. One single cell, probably a damaged mesothelial cell, shows nonspecific staining by the dye. (Magnification × 83.)

PLATE 13.   A section of primary mammary carcinoma shows a clone of ER-positive and a clone of ER-negative cancer cells growing next to each other with a sharp demarcation between the two. (Magnification × 83.)

PLATE 14.   Benign intraductal papillomatous hyperplasia in a female breast. Note a rather uniform degree of estrogen binding activity in the cytoplasm of the epithelial cells. (Magnification × 83.)

PLATE 15.   Intraductal papillary carcinoma showing one roll of ER-positive malignant epithelial cells next to a mass of morphologically similar, but ER-negative cancer cells. (Magnification × 83.)

PLATE 16.   Intraductal papillary carcinoma in the same tumor shown in Plate 15. Note a strip of ER-positive benign epithelial cells being compressed by a mass of encroaching cancerous cells within the same duct. There is a distinct difference in size between the benign epithelial cells and the cancer cells. (Magnification × 83.)

PLATE 17.   Lobular carcinoma *in situ* showing ER-positive and ER-negative cancer cells growing side by side within the same terminal duct. (Magnification × 83.)

PLATE 18.   Lobular carcinoma *in situ* showing terminal ducts distended by clones of ER-positive cancer cells as well as ER-negative cancer cells next to each other. No compressing effects are recognized. (Magnification × 83.)

closely in time sequence. The synthesis of both estrogen receptor and progesterone receptor in the rat uterus has been known to increase after injections of estrogens.[48] The advantage of incorporating a fluorescent progesterone conjugate in the histochemical reagent is that it may help to ascertain the ER-positive cancer cells being observed are, indeed, functionally responding to estrogenic stimulation by synthesizing an intracellular product — progesterone receptor.[4] Necrotic cell debris tend to bind one type of the reagent, but not the other (Plates 4 and 5). Among the undamaged tissue structures, myelinated peripheral nerves often bind both fluorescent estrogen and progesterone conjugates nonspecifically, probably because they are rich in myelin that may also have a high affinity for steroid compounds (Plates 6 to 8).

It cannot be overemphasized that a surgical pathologist who is actively involved in diagnostic tissue pathology should examine the histochemical preparations. It is sometimes difficult enough to recognize human mammary carcinoma cells in a regular frozen section stained with hematoxylin and eosin and viewed with a light microscope. At least some of the poor results reported to be produced by the histochemical assays might have been attributed to an incorrect interpretation of a cancer preparation. The ER-positive benign epithelial cells in foci of sclerosing adenosis, distorted hyperplastic ductal epithelial cells, and eosinophil leukocytes may be mistaken for cancer cells in the fluorescence microscope by those who only maintain a casual contact with diagnostic tissue pathology or not at all. Even a seasoned diagnostician must be aware of the pitfall that crushed or necrotic cancer cells may absorb fluorescent dyes nonspecifically, and should be discounted during examination. This type of nonspecific fluorescence occurs often in the cancer cells at the margin of a section where crushing artifacts are most evident (Plate 9). Surgical clamps and the teeth of forceps can produce similar results.

## B. Malignant Effusions

A diagnostic problem arises when a female patient develops a malignant pleural effusion containing adenocarcinoma cells of unknown origin. The most common primary lesion in such a situation is either a pulmonary or a mammary occult tumor; but it is often difficult to decide which one is correct based on cytologic studies of the cells in effusions alone. Under these circumstances, the pathologist is often requested to use all measures at his or her disposal to render a best presumptive diagnosis because of the potential difference in therapeutic and prognostic implications involved. A cytochemical ER assay may play an important role since the diagnosis of a mammary cancer can be established if the cancer cells are found to be ER-positive, although a negative result does not help to solve the problem.

The technology as to what is the best way to perform a cytochemical assay for malignant effusions is still at a stage of being further refined. At the time of this writing, the most reliable method seems to use cryostat frozen sections of a cell block. The section will then be treated and stained in a manner similar to that for tissue sections. A packed cell pellet of about 0.5 mℓ in volume derived from an aliquot of the usually bloody specimen is resuspended in a phosphate buffered saline, pH 7.4, in a 15-mℓ conical polystyrene centrifuge tube. After the supernatant is decanted, the pellet is frozen at $-70°C$ for a few minutes. The centrifuge tube is then cracked open with a pair of pliers near the conical tip to release the frozen cell pellet intact. The latter is immediately embedded in an OTC medium sideways on a metal chuck for cryostat sectioning. The red blood cells are usually settled in the bottom layer of the pellet; the second and the third layers are formed by the lymphocytes and cancer cells mixed with mesothelial cells, respectively (Plates 10 to 12).

Several unsuccessful attempts have been made to stain the ER-positive cancer cells in suspension, as described for trypsinized MCF-7 cells.[45] There are also difficulties in using cryostat frozen sections of cell blocks of MCF-7 cells for ER assay. Perhaps the cytoskeleton which the intracellular estrogen receptors are associated with is different in these two forms of malignant cells. Needless to say, the most difficult task in dealing with malignant effusions is to recognize the cancer cells with fluorescence microscopy. It needs a large number of cancer cells in the specimen for the technique to be successful. Again, it must be emphasized that any cells mechanically damaged may take in fluorescent dyes nonspecifically. A section of a cell block containing only isolated fluorescent cells should be regarded as ER-negative.

## C. Biology of Potentially Hormone-Responsive Cancers

Based on correlations between ER protein assay and the clinical response, it has been found that in most ER-positive breast cancers hormonal manipulation only induces partial and short-term remissions. Eventually, almost all cancers under treatment progress to an autonomous condition.[4] It is not clear whether the ratio of ER-positive to ER-negative cancer cells changes significantly during the course of hormonal therapy. Not infrequently, a breast cancer contains clones of ER-positive and ER-negative cancer cells with a sharp demarcation between the clones (Plate 13). One simplistic hypothesis would be that hormonal manipulation affects the growth of the ER-positive cancer cells only. In the end when the treatment was no longer effective, the ER-negative cells became prevalent in the cancer cell population. A histochemical approach can provide a means to study the cellular composition of the heterogeneous cancer and may generate new information in this respect.

Another interesting question is how and why breast cancer cells become ER-positive or ER-negative from the start. Assuming that all infiltrating cancers begin as an intraductal or intralobular growth at one point, it seems logical that one should approach this problem when the cancerous lesion is still at a preinvasive stage. Such an endeavor can only be undertaken using a histochemical technique.

After a fair number of histochemical preparations of human breast specimens with intraductal epithelial proliferative lesions having been examined, the results seem to indicate the following:

1.   The epithelial cells in an unquestionably benign intraductal papillomatous growth usually show a rather uniform degree of cytoplasmic estrogen binding activity (Plate 14). If there is a cellular heterogeneity, the hyperplastic ER-positive cells tend to be dispersed more or less evenly or in a random fashion among the ER-negative cells.

2.   The intraductal papillary carcinomas often have foci of ER-positive and ER-negative cancer cells, apparently growing in clones next to each other (Plate 15). One can find an occasional remnant of benign ER-positive epithelial cells being compressed by the encroaching cancerous mass which is mostly composed of ER-negative cells (Plate 16). This phenomenon in which one clone of ER-negative cells appears to proliferate at the expense of the adjacent ER-positive epithelium within the same mammary duct has been only observed in obviously malignant lesions, and not in benign papillomas; therefore, it seems that if present, this encroachment phenomenon may serve as a potential criterion to differentiate a malignant lesion from a benign papillary growth.

3.   The noninfiltrating solid or comedo carcinomas are largely composed of ER-negative cancer cells.[8]

4.   The cancer cells in lobular carcinomas *in situ* seem to be heterogeneous in ER positivity right from the early stage of development, characterized by an apparently simultaneous proliferation of both ER-positive and ER-negative cancer cells in the same terminal ducts. This process leads to a heterogeneous cellular composition even in a small segment of a lobule where individual ER-positive and ER-negative cancer cells may grow side by side (Plate 17), or form small clones distending different terminal ducts within the same lobule (Plate 18). It is of interest to note that when the ER-positive and the ER-negative cancer cells proliferate simultaneously in the same terminal duct, no encroachment effect has been observed.

**D. Applications in Other Cancers**

As the criteria for the histochemical assay of estrogen receptors in breast cancer are being established, there is a natural temptation to expand the application of this procedure to study other potentially hormone-sensitive cancers, such as those of endometrium, ovary, and prostate. However, it is advisable that a separate set of cytochemical criteria be established to determine the receptor positivity for the tumors of each of these organs. Overextrapolation of the data derived from studies of breast cancer cells in these other situations should be avoided. For one reason, the number of receptor sites even in the normal cells of these organs may differ from those in the mammary glands. This author has studied only a limited number of cases of endometrial carcinoma, and found them to be highly heterogeneous in cytoplasmic estrogen receptor level. The cancer cells are largely ER-negative. Even when positive, the intensity of intracellular fluorescence is far below that observed in the ER-positive breast cancer cells. According to a recent report by two investigators,[49] the cancer cells of the well-differentiated adenocarcinomas of the endometrium may contain a higher number of estrogen binding sites than those in a less-differentiated ones. The undifferentiated tumors may have almost no ER-positive cancer cells.

In applying this technique to the study of prostatic carcinomas, a similar cancer cell heterogeneity and correlation of ER levels with the degrees of tumor differentiation has been observed. To further complicate the situation, effects of cauterization that are often evident at the periphery of the prostatic tissue chips may cause severe cellular damages, resulting in loss of the cytoplasmic estrogen binding activity and appearance of a nonspecific nuclear staining.

Cytoplasmic estrogen binding in ovarian cancers, similar to that in mammary carcinoma, is also highly heterogeneous. The progress in this area is hindered by the limited number of cases available in a general hospital and by the notorious variety of the cancers of the ovary.

## V. CONCLUDING REMARKS

The value of a histochemical method for identifying human cancer cells rich in estrogen receptors has been increasingly recognized by biochemists, pathologists, and clinicians because of its simplicity and its potential to provide an alternative means to study the estrogen receptors that truly represent a function of the cancer cell population. The technique described in this chapter has been in wide use for 3 to 5 years in many laboratories. Now there seems to have been a volume of data to indicate that the intracellular estrogen binding substance so demonstrated does satisfy the criteria defined for estrogen receptors, although one may still question whether it may be a mixture of the type I and type II binding sites; but the binding activity in the cancer cells is highly unlikely to be caused by the so-called type III binders. Nevertheless, it must be emphasized that due precautions must be taken in the handling of specimens and in interpretation of the histochemical preparations in order to obtain a valid result. At least some of the failures to obtain a satisfactory correlation between the histochemical assay and other known parameters of the human breast cancer may have been due to inappropriate storage of the specimens and possibly due to the use of a histochemical reagent of uncertain quality.[50] As pointed out by one group of investigators recently, neither the histochemical nor the biochemical method can be regarded as an easy, routine technique, and previous studies in which comparisons have failed to show a good correlation between cytochemical and quantitative biochemical assays may have been influenced by such considerations.[23]

As this technique is designed to detect a function of the cancer cells, no one else but a pathologist familiar with diagnostic cancer pathology should interpret the histochemical preparations. The examining pathologist should realize, also, that there must be numerous types of estrogen target cells in a microscopic tissue section, considering the wide spectrum of physiologic influence of estrogens on the human body. These target cells may contain varying amounts of estrogen receptors and respond to estrogenic stimulation with different magnitudes and in different manners. It is conceivable that because of its relatively low sensitivity as compared to various radioactive isotope binding assays, the fluorescent histochemical technique can detect only the target cells with an exceptionally high estrogen binding capacity against a background of other cell types that may still contain many estrogen target cells in the broad sense. The incorporation of a progesterone histochemical reagent labeled with a fluorescent dye other than FITC has been found helpful to the pathologist to identify the epithelial cells which react to estrogenic stimulation by synthesizing a cytoplasmic progesterone receptor. It seems that in the human breast only the epithelial cells of the mammary ducts or carcinomas have this potential. To what extent this histochemical technique is useful in the practice of diagnostic pathology, for example, in selecting hormone-responsive cancers for hormonal therapy and in studying the pathology of different kinds of proliferative lesions in the breast will depend on large-scale collaborative studies involving interested surgical pathologists and their clinical colleagues. The initial experience of several research groups can be found elsewhere in this volume.

## ACKNOWLEDGMENTS

The author wishes to express his appreciation to Ms. Doris Barclay for skilled photographic assistance, and to Miss Marilyn Weed for secretarial assistance.

## REFERENCES

1. **Jensen, E. V., Block, G. E., Smith, S., Kyser, K., and DeSombre, E. R.,** Estrogen receptors and breast cancer response to adrenalectomy, *Natl. Cancer Inst. Monogr.,* 34, 55, 1971.
2. **McGuire, W. L., Vollmer, E. P., and Carbone, P. P., Eds.,** *Estrogen Receptors in Human Breast Cancer,* Raven Press, New York, 1975.
3. **Heuson, J. C., Longeval, E., Mattheiem, W. H., Deboel, M. C., Sylvester, R. J., and Leclercq, G.,** Significance of quantitative assessment of estrogen receptors for endocrine therapy in advanced breast cancer, *Cancer,* 39, 1971, 1977.
4. **McGuire, W. L., Horwitz, K. B., Pearson, O. H., and Segaloff, A.,** Current status of estrogen and progesterone receptors in breast cancer, *Cancer,* 39, 2934, 1977.
5. **Nenci, I., Beccati, M. D., Piffanelli, A., and Lanza, G.,** Detection and dynamic localisation of estradiol-receptor complexes in intact target cells by immunofluorescence technique, *J. Steroid Biochem.,* 7, 505, 1976.
6. **Pertschuk, L. P.,** Detection of estrogen binding in human mammary carcinoma by immunofluorescence: a new technic utilizing the binding hormone in a polymerized state, *Res. Commun. Chem. Pathol. Pharmacol.,* 14, 771, 1976.
7. **Lee, S. H.,** Cytochemical study of estrogen receptor in human mammary cancer, *Am. J. Clin. Pathol.,* 70, 197, 1978.
8. **Lee, S. H.,** Cancer cell estrogen receptor mammary carcinoma, *Cancer,* 44, 1, 1979.
9. **Lee, S. H.,** The histochemistry of estrogen receptors, *Histochemistry,* 71, 491, 1981.
10. **Lee, S. H.,** Uterine epithelial and eosinophil estrogen receptors in rats during the estrous cycle, *Histochemistry,* 74, 443, 1982.
11. **Lee, S. H.,** Estrogen-primed immature rat uterus — a tissue control for histochemical estrogen receptor assay, *Am. J. Clin. Pathol.,* 79, 484, 1983.

12. **Lee, S. H.,** Validity of a histochemical estrogen receptor assay, supported by the observation of a cellular response to steroid manipulation, *J. Histochem. Cytochem.,* in press.

13. **Lee, S. H.,** Histochemical study of estrogen receptors in the rat uterus with a hydrophilic fluorescent estradiol conjugate, in *Localization of Putative Steroid Receptors,* Vol. 1, Pertschuk, L. P. and Lee, S. H., Eds., CRC Press, Boca Raton, Fla., in press.

14. **Fetisof, F., Lansac, J., and Arbeilli-Brassart, B.,** Mise en évidence des récepteurs de l'oestradiol et de la progestérone sur préparations histologiques, *Ann. Anat. Pathol. Paris,* 25, 201, 1980.

15. **Paulsen, S. M., Johansen, P., Rasmussen, K. S., and Mygind, H.,** Histochemical demonstration of oestrogen receptors in cancer of the breast, *Ugeskr. Laeg.,* 143, 3119, 1981.

16. **Tominaga, T., Kitamura, M., Saito, T., Itoh, I., and Takikawa, H.,** Comparative histochemical and biochemical assays of estrogen receptors in breast cancer patients, *Gann,* 72, 60, 1981.

17. **Van Marle, J., Lindeman, J., Ariëns, A. Th., Labruyere, W., and Van Weeren-Kramer, J.,** Estrogen receptors in human breast cancer. I. Specificity of the histochemical localization of estrogen receptors using an estrogen-albumin FITC complex, *Virchows Arch. (Cell Pathol.),* 40, 17, 1982.

18. **Eusebi, V., Cerasoli, P. T., Guidelli-Guidi, S., Grilli, S., Bussolati, G., and Azzopardi, J. G.,** A two-stage immunocytochemical method for oestrogen receptor analysis: correlation with morphological parameters of breast carcinomas, *Tumori,* 67, 315, 1981.

19. **Hanna, W., Ryder, D. E., and Mobbs, B. G.,** Cellular localization of estrogen binding sites in human breast cancer, *Am. J. Clin. Pathol.,* 77, 391, 1982.

20. **Jacobs, S. R., Wolfson, W. L., Cheng, L., and Lewin, K. J.,** Cytochemical and competitive protein binding assays for estrogen receptor in breast disease, *Cancer,* 51, 1621, 1983.

21. **O'Connell, M. D. and Said, J. W.,** Estrogen receptors in carcinoma of the breast. A comparison of the dextran-coated charcoal, immunofluorescent, and immunoperoxidase technique, *Am. J. Clin. Pathol.,* 80, 1, 1983.

22. **Yao, X., Meng, X., Chen, P., and Mei, Z.,** Histochemical estrogen receptor assay for selecting stage III breast cancers for combined chemohormonal therapy, *Lab. Invest.,* 48, 95, 1983.

23. **Furnival, C. M., Chong, K. C., Watson, L. R., and Visona, A.,** Fluorescent cytochemical oestrogen receptor assay: is it valid in breast cancer?, *Br. J. Surg.,* 70, 457, 1983.

24. **Lee, S. H.,** Sex steroid hormone receptors in mammary carcinoma, in *Diagnostic Immunohistochemistry,* DeLellis, R. A., Ed., Masson Publishing, New York, 1981, 149.

25. **Lee, S. H.,** Hydrophilic macromolecules of steroid derivatives for the detection of cancer cell receptors, *Cancer,* 46, 2825, 1980.

26. **Jensen, E. V. and Jacobson, H. I.,** Basic guides to the mechanism of estrogen action, *Recent Prog. Horm. Res.,* 18, 387, 1962.

27. **Gorski, J., Toft, D., Shyamala, G., Smith, D., and Notides, A.,** Hormone receptors: studies on the interaction of estrogen with the uterus, *Recent Prog. Horm. Res.,* 24, 45, 1968.

28. **Jensen, E. V. and DeSombre, E. R.,** Mechanism of action of the female sex hormones, *Annu. Rev. Biochem.,* 41, 203, 1972.

29. **McCarty, K. S., Jr., Woodard, B. H., Nichols, D. E., Wilkinson, W., and McCarty, K. S., Sr.,** Comparison of biochemical and histochemical techniques for estrogen receptor analyses in mammary carcinoma, *Cancer,* 46, 2842, 1980.

30. **Panko, W. B., Mattioli, C. A., and Wheeler, T. M.,** Lack of correlation of a histochemical method for estrogen receptor analysis results, *Cancer,* 49, 2148, 1982.

31. **Chamness, G. C., Mercer, W. D., and McGuire, W. L.,** Are histochemical methods for estrogen receptor valid?, *J. Histochem. Cytochem.,* 28, 792, 1980.

32. **Chamness, G. C. and McGuire, W. L.,** Questions about histochemical methods for steroid receptors, *Arch. Pathol. Lab. Med.,* 106, 53, 1982.

33. **DeSombre, E. R., Carbone, P. P., Jensen, E. V., McGuire, W. L., Wells, S. A., Jr., Wittliff, J. L., and Lipsett, M. B.,** Steroid receptors in breast cancer (report of a consensus-development meeting, NIH, June, 1979), *N. Engl. J. Med.,* 301, 1011, 1979.

34. **King, R. J. B., Barnes, D. M., Hawkins, R. A., Leake, R. E., Maynard, P. V., Millis, R. M., and Roberts, M. M.,** Measurement of oestrogen receptors by five institutions on common tissue samples, in *Steroid Receptor Assays in Human Breast Tumours: Methodological and Clinical Aspects,* King, R. J. B., Ed., Alpha Omega Publishing, Cardiff, 1979, 7.

35. **Oxley, D. K.,** Hormone receptors in breast cancer, analytic accuracy of contemporary assays, *Arch. Pathol. Lab. Med.,* 108, 20, 1984.

36. **Sarfaty, G. A., Nash, A. R., and Keightley, D. D., Eds.,** *Estrogen Receptor Assays in Breast Cancer, Laboratory Discrepancies and Quality Assurance,* Masson Publishing, New York, 1981.

37. **Feherty, P., Robertson, D. M., Waynforth, H. B., and Kellie, A. E.,** Changes in the concentration of high-affinity oestradiol receptors in rat uterine supernatant preparations during the oestrous cycle, pseudopregnancy, pregnancy, maturation, and after ovariectomy, *Biochem. J.,* 120, 837, 1970.

38. **Lee, C. and Jacobson, H. I.,** Uterine estrogen receptor in rats during pubescence and the estrous cycle, *Endocrinology,* 88, 596, 1971.

39. **Kielhorn, J. and Hughes, A.,** Variations in uterine cytosolic oestrogen and progesterone receptor levels during the rat estrous cycle, *Acta Endocrinol.,* 86, 842, 1977.

40. **Clark, J. H. and Peck, E. J., Jr.,** Steroid hormone receptors: basic principles and measurement, in *Receptors and Hormone Action,* Vol. 1, O'Malley, B. W. and Birnbaumer, L., Eds., Academic Press, New York, 1977, 383.

41. **DeGoeij, A. F. P. M., Volleberg, M. P. W., Hondius, G. E., Frederik, P. M., and Bosman, F. T.,** Quantitative estrogen receptor assay on frozen sections using radiolabeled estradiol, *J. Steroid Biochem.,* 19, 100S, 1983.

42. **Clark, J. H., Markaverich, B., Upchurch, S., Eriksson, H., Hardin, J. W., and Peck, E. J., Jr.,** Heterogeneity of estrogen binding sites: relationship to estrogen receptors and estrogen responses, *Recent Prog. Horm. Res.,* 36, 89, 1980.

43. **Eriksson, H. A., Hardin, J. W., Markaverich, B., Upchurch, S., and Clark, J. H.,** Estrogen binding in the rat uterus: heterogeneity of sites and relation to uterotrophic response, *J. Steroid Biochem.,* 12, 121, 1980.

44. **Goldstein, L.,** Kinetic behavior of immobilized enzyme systems, *Methods Enzymol.,* 44, 397, 1976.

45. **Benz, C., Wiznitzer, I., and Lee, S. H.,** Flow cytometric analysis of fluorescent estrogen binding in cancer cell suspensions, in *Localization of Putative Steroid Receptors,* Vol. 1, Pertschuk, L. P. and Lee, S. H., Eds., CRC Press, Boca Raton, Fla., in press.

46. **Lee, S. H.,** Prospects for histochemical assay of steroid receptors, in *Endocrine Relationships in Breast Cancer,* Vol. 5, Stoll, B. A., Ed., William Heinemann Medical Book, London, 1982, 144.

47. **Lee, S. H.,** Cellular estrogen and progesterone receptors in mammary carcinoma, *Am. J. Clin. Pathol.,* 73, 323, 1980.

48. **Clark, J. H., Hsueh, A. J. W., and Peck, E. G., Jr.,** Regulation of estrogen receptor replenishment by progesterone, *Ann. N.Y. Acad. Sci.,* 286, 161, 1977.

49. **Grille, J. and Albert, P.,** Neue morphologische Gesichtspunkte des Endometriumkarzinoms, *Arch. Gynecol.,* 235, 186, 1983.

50. **McCarty, K. S., Jr., Hiatt, K. B., Budwit, D. A., Cox, E. B., Leight, G., Reintgen, D., Georgiade, G., McCarty, K. S., Sr., and Siegler, H. F.,** Clinical response to hormone therapy correlated with estrogen receptor analyses, *Arch. Pathol. Lab. Med.,* 108, 24, 1984.

Chapter 4

# HISTOCHEMICAL SEX STEROID HORMONE RECEPTOR ASSAY AND TREATMENT OF BREAST CANCER IN CHINESE PATIENTS

**Peizhen Chen, Xianyun Yao, Zhijia Mei, and Xiangin Meng**

## TABLE OF CONTENTS

I.    Introduction...................................................................52

II.   Materials and Methods.......................................................52
     A.    Histochemical Steroid Hormone Receptor Assay.........................52
     B.    Clinical and Pathological Materials.....................................52
     C.    Assessment of Therapeutic Efficacy....................................53

III.  Results.....................................................................53
     A.    Frequency of HR-Rich Breast Cancers ................................54
     B.    Status of Menstruation of the Patient and the HR Value ...............54
     C.    Tumor HR Status and Age of the Patient...............................54
     D.    HR Status and Histological Types of Tumors .........................54
     E.    Variability of Tumor HR Status in the Same Patient ...................56
     F.    Survival Rate and HR Status in Advanced Cases.......................56
     G.    Endocrine Therapy in Reducing HR-Rich Tumor Size .................57

IV.  Discussion .................................................................57

References.......................................................................59

# I. INTRODUCTION

As one of the most common malignancies in women, the incidence of breast cancer in China is only second to that of carcinoma of the uterine cervix. With the development of methods of hormone receptor assay and their clinical application, most practicing oncologists have classified breast cancers into two categories, namely, the steroid hormone receptor-positive and the steroid hormone receptor-negative; and the hormone receptor status of the tumor is regarded as an important parameter in assessment of the patient's condition, the planning of treatment protocol, and the prediction of response to endocrine therapy. However, to obtain the most favorable therapeutic response to endocrine therapy, considerations should also be given to other prognostic factors, including clinical and pathological features of the cancer. Several authors have examined the relationship between pathological features of the breast cancer and the steroid hormone receptor levels, but the results are rather controversial.

In China, preliminary exploration of many new diagnostic laboratory techniques is only beginning, and neither the biochemical nor the histochemical method for tumor receptor assay has been established in clinical practice. This chapter represents a preliminary report on the application of Lee's histochemical method[1-4] of hormone receptor assay for the study of the pathology and the clinical course of the breast cancers in 145 patients.

# II. MATERIALS AND METHODS

## A. Histochemical Steroid Hormone Receptor Assay

From July 1980 to September 1983, a fluorescent histochemical assay of cytoplasmic estrogen receptor and/or progesterone receptor was carried out on 256 fresh specimens surgically excised for diagnostic or for therapeutic purposes; among them 162 from 145 patients proved to be malignant histologically. Unfixed serial cryostat frozen sections were cut from each specimen, air-dried, and stained with a macromolecular hydrophilic fluorescent steroid conjugate containing $2 \times 10^{-4}$ $M$ bound estradiol or progesterone derivative[1,3] (a gift from Dr. S. H. Lee, Department of Pathology, Hospital of St. Raphael, New Haven, Conn.). These sections were examined with a fluorescence microscope equipped with filters specific for fluorescein and for rhodamine excitation. The cells which manifested apple-green or orange-red fluorescence were considered positive for estrogen receptor or progesterone receptor, respectively.

The intensity of fluorescence of the receptor-positive benign ductal epithelial cells was used as the standard for comparison. The cancer cells that fluoresced as intensely as or more than the benign ductal epithelial cells were considered sex steroid receptor positive. The stroma generally showed slight nonspecific fluorescence only. The necrotic cancer cells and the lymphocytes which infiltrated the tumor tissue showed no fluorescence. For each tumor, the percentage of steroid receptor-positive cancer cells in the malignant epithelial cell population was estimated and recorded by a surgical pathologist.[5,6] However, for therapeutic purposes the cancers were divided arbitrarily into two categories. The tumors with less than 50% of the infiltrating cancer cells showing cytoplasmic fluorescence were classified as hormone receptor-poor, those with 50% or more cancer cells fluorescent as hormone receptor-rich.

## B. Clinical and Pathological Materials

During this period of study, 141 women and 4 men with breast cancer were admitted for treatment and their tumors were assessed for cytoplasmic hormone receptor. There was a post-treatment follow-up for 9 to 36 months in 99.5% of the patients.

The breast cancers were classified according to 1982 WHO Histological Typing of Breast Tumors.[7]

The clinical staging system for carcinoma of the breast adopted by the International Union Against Cancer in 1958 and 1977 was used to classify the patients into three groups, namely, early ($T_{1-2}N_{0-1}M_0$), intermediate ($T_{2-3}N_{0-1}M_0$), and advanced ($T_3N_2M_0$). The advanced group also included those cases in terminal stage ($T_4$).

Radical mastectomy was the primary operation performed for the advanced and intermediate cases. The early cases received modified radical mastectomy or simple mastectomy. A simple or partial mastectomy was also performed in some patients with advanced disease.

Radiotherapy was given to the patients with evidence of lymphatic metastases. The patients who had undergone radical mastectomy were treated by deep X-ray radiation to the supra- and infraclavicular, medial mammary, and infraaxillary regions. The patients who had undergone modified radical mastectomy or simple mastectomy were radiated by a Cobalt-60 unit (THERATRON-80®); the radiation covered four fields, namely, the chest wall, infraaxillary, supra-, and infraclavicular regions. In some cases, a fifth field, namely, the medial mammary region, was also irradiated.

Sixty-nine patients were treated by a combined endocrine and polychemotherapy. Of these, 25 patients were given preoperative chemotherapeutic medication, including 1 mg of vincristine, 250 to 500 mg of 5-fluorouracil, and 200 to 400 mg of cyclophosphamide once a week for 8 to 10 weeks; the other 44 patients were given 1 mg of vincristine, 500 mg of 5-fluorouracil, and 400 mg of cyclophosphamide administered once a week for 5 to 10 weeks. The types of endocrine therapy consisted of bilateral oophorectomy for the premenopausal and perimenopausal (within 5 years after the last menstrual period) women, and medications which included 50 mg of testosterone propionate every other day, 10 mg of tamoxifen twice a day, or 4 mg of diethylstilbestrol (DES) twice or thrice a day to the postmenopausal. When the patients presented with an advanced disease that was considered not suitable for a primary resection, a combined endocrine and chemotherapy was first instituted. After the tumors had reduced by more than 50% in size, the patients then underwent simple mastectomy or radiotherapy. Thirty-two patients were not given endocrine therapy either because it was medically contraindicated or because the patient refused to receive hormones.

## C. Assessment of Therapeutic Efficacy

The following criteria were used for the assessment of response to therapy:

1. **Complete response**: disappearance of all signs of the disease without appearance of new lesions during the 9- to 36-month period of observation
2. **Partial response**: decrease in measurable tumor nodules in size by 50% or more, bone metastases stationary for at least 3 months, disappearance or remission of lung metastases, while no new lesions appearing and no old lesions progressing for a period of at least 6 months
3. **Failure**: no change or increase in measurable tumor nodules, appearance of new lesions, or death with spreading diseases

## III. RESULTS

In our experience, all cancer cells which were found to be positive for cytoplasmic estrogen receptor also contained cytoplasmic progesterone receptor. Therefore, the number of estrogen receptor-positive and the number of progesterone receptor-positive cancer cells in each tumor were identical, and the tumor cells were generally referred to as sex steroid hormone receptor (HR)-positive cells. The tumors containing 50% or more of receptor-positive cells in their cancer cell population were referred to as being HR-rich and the tumors in which the receptor-negative cancer cells exceeded 50% were arbitrarily classified as receptor-poor.

**Table 1**
**HR STATUS AND STAGE OF BREAST CANCER IN 141**
**CHINESE WOMEN**

| Cancer cells HR + (%) | Stage of disease | | | | | |
|---|---|---|---|---|---|---|
| | Early | | Intermediate | | Advanced | |
| | No. of cases | % | No. of cases | % | No. of cases | % |
| >90 | 3 | 7.0 | 3 | 10.0 | 6 | 8.8 |
| 80—89 | 0 | 0 | 3 | 10.0 | 7 | 10.3 |
| 70—79 | 3 | 7.0 | 2 | 6.7 | 9 | 13.2 |
| 60—69 | 2 | 4.7 | 2 | 6.7 | 3 | 4.4 |
| 50—59 | 4 | 9.3 | 2 | 6.7 | 13 | 19.1 |
| 40—49 | 1 | 2.3 | 0 | 0 | 1 | 1.5 |
| 30—39 | 13 | 30.2 | 5 | 16.6 | 19 | 28.0 |
| 20—29 | 4 | 9.3 | 4 | 13.3 | 2 | 2.9 |
| 10—19 | 10 | 23.2 | 9 | 30.0 | 8 | 11.8 |
| 0—9 | 3 | 7.0 | | | | |
| Total | 43 | 100 | 30 | 100 | 68 | 100 |

## A. Frequency of HR-Rich Breast Cancers

Among 162 cancerous specimens which were obtained from the primary sites, metastatic lesions in region lymph nodes, or recurrent nodules in the chest wall, 72 tumors (44.4%) were HR-rich and 90 (55.6%) were HR-poor. The latter group also included four HR-poor male breast cancers.

Table 1 shows the relationship between the HR status and the disease stage of 141 female breast cancers. Although the overall number of the HR-rich tumors constituted 44% (62 cases) of the total, the percentage dropped to 28% in the early cases. The HR-rich cancers amounted to 44.1 and 55.8% in the patients with intermediate and advanced stage of the disease, respectively. Thus, the patients who presented with a more advanced stage of disease were more likely to have an HR-rich cancer than those with an early disease.

## B. Status of Menstruation of the Patient and the HR Value

As shown in Table 2, both the HR-rich and the HR-poor cancers were encountered most commonly in perimenopausal patients, constituting 62 and 59%, respectively. A similar incidence was obtained with a control group of 117 patients whose tumors were not evaluated for HR status.

## C. Tumor HR Status and Age of the Patient

Attempts were made to determine whether there was a relationship between the HR status of breast cancer and the age of the patient. The results summarized in Table 3 showed that there was no significant difference in the patients' age distribution among HR-rich, HR-poor, and the unassayed tumors. The youngest patient was 28 and the oldest 74, with the largest number of cases between 40 and 49 years of age in all three groups.

## D. HR Status and Histological Types of Tumors

Of the 162 cancerous specimens studied, 123 were classified as infiltrating ductal carcinomas, 8 medullary carcinomas, 4 infiltrating lobular carcinomas, 4 mucinous carcinomas, 3 papillary carcinomas, and 1 Paget's disease of the breast. In addition, there were 19

**Table 2**
**THE DISTRIBUTION OF HR-RICH AND HR-POOR TUMORS IN DIFFERENT MENSTRUAL GROUPS**

|  | HR-rich | | HR-poor | | HR-rich cases (%) |
|---|---|---|---|---|---|
|  | No. | % | No. | % |  |
| Premenopausal | 12 | 19 | 15 | 19.2 | 44.4 |
| Perimenopausal | 39 | 62 | 46 | 59.0 | 46.4 |
| Postmenopausal | 12 | 19 | 17 | 21.8 | 41.4 |
| Total | 63 | 100 | 78 | 100 |  |

**Table 3**
**HR STATUS OF BREAST CANCER AND THE AGE OF THE PATIENTS**

| Age (years) | HR-rich | | HR-poor | | Unassayed | |
|---|---|---|---|---|---|---|
|  | No. | % | No. | % | No. | % |
| <30 | 1 | 1.6 | 0 | 0 | 3 | 2.5 |
| 30—39 | 13 | 20.6 | 16 | 19.5 | 23 | 19.7 |
| 40—49 | 28 | 44.5 | 32 | 39.0 | 49 | 41.9 |
| 50—59 | 16 | 25.4 | 20 | 24.4 | 30 | 25.6 |
| 60— | 5 | 7.9 | 14 | 17.1 | 12 | 10.3 |
| Total | 63 | 100 | 82 | 100 | 117 | 100 |

**Table 4**
**CORRELATION BETWEEN THE HR STATUS AND HISTOPATHOLOGICAL TYPES OF BREAST CARCINOMA**

| Histopathologic types | No. of cases | HR-rich | | HR-poor | |
|---|---|---|---|---|---|
|  |  | No. | % | No. | % |
| Infiltrating ductal | 123 | 52 | 42.3 | 71[a] | 57.7 |
| Infiltrating lobular | 4 | 2 | 50 | 2 | 50 |
| Medullary | 8 | 4 | 50 | 4 | 50 |
| Mucinous | 4 | 3 | 75 | 1 | 25 |
| Papillary | 3 | 0 | 0 | 3 | 100 |
| Paget's disease | 1 |  |  | 1 |  |
| Unclassified | 19 | 11 | 57.9 | 8 | 42.1 |
| Total | 162 | 72 |  | 90 |  |

[a]   Including four male cases.

unclassified carcinomas. Among the 72 HR-rich tumors, 52 were infiltrating ductal carcinomas, 4 medullary carcinomas, 3 mucinous carcinomas, 2 infiltrating lobular carcinomas, and 11 unclassified. In all three cases of papillary carcinomas, and one case of Paget's disease, the HR receptor-positive cancer cell counts were found to be of a low level (Table 4).

**Table 5**
**CHANGES OF HR LEVELS IN FOUR CASES OF**
**BREAST CANCER**

| Patient identification | HR-positive cancer cells (%) | | Interval between two assays (months) |
|---|---|---|---|
| | 1st Assay | 2nd Assay | |
| Sh | <10 | 50 | 12 |
| Su | 50 | 70 | 18 |
| He | 90 | 70 | 22 |
| Hu | 90 | 30 | 9 |

**Table 6**
**HR STATUS OF BREAST CANCER AND THE OUTCOME**
**OF DISEASE IN 70 PATIENTS**

| Outcome | Stage of disease | | | |
|---|---|---|---|---|
| | $T_3N_2M_0$ | | $T_4N_3M_1$ | |
| | HR-rich cases | HR-poor cases | HR-rich cases | HR-poor cases |
| Survival without recurrence | 14 | 9 | 8 | 1 |
| Survival with recurrence | 3 | 3 | 0 | 0 |
| Death | 4 | 10 | 10 | 8 |
| Survival (%) | 81.0 | 54.5 | 44.4 | 11.1 |

## E. Variability of Tumor HR Status in the Same Patient

In 11 patients whose tumor contained receptor-positive cancer cells, we had the opportunity to examine the HR status of the primary cancer and the metastatic lesions in lymph nodes at the same time, and found an almost identical percentage of receptor-positive cancer cells in the primary and second lesions in eight cases (72.7%). In the other three cases, two had a lower percentage of receptor-positive cancer cells in the metastatic lesions than in the primary. In one case, there was a higher receptor-positive cell count in the lymph nodes than in the primary.

In four cases, the HR assays of the primary and the recurrent lesions were performed at different times with a 9- to 22-month interval. The changes of HR levels of the tumor appeared to be irregular; the receptor-positive cell count was found to increase in two of the cases and decrease in the other two during the course of the disease (Table 5).

## F. Survival Rate and HR Status in Advanced Cases

In order to test the value of the histochemical HR assay in predicting the clinical course in terms of survival, 70 patients with advanced breast cancer were further divided into two groups, namely, those of stage $T_3N_2M_0$ and those with stage $T_4N_3M_1$ disease, and followed up for 9 to 36 months. During this period, the patients with HR-rich tumors at stage $T_3N_2M_0$ had a survival rate of 81.0%, whereas those with HR-poor cancers had a rate of 54.5%. A survival rate of 44.4 and 11.1% was observed in patients with terminal, stage $T_4N_3M_1$ disease, also indicating that the patients with HR-rich tumors tended to live longer (Table 6), with a survival rate four times that for the patients with HR-poor tumors.

## G. Endocrine Therapy in Reducing HR-Rich Tumor Size

During this period of study, we used an initial combined endocrine and chemotherapy in 20 late-stage breast cancer patients with HR-rich tumors, in whom surgical treatment was considered unfavorable. The lesions in 18 of the 20 cases showed a striking partial response and eventually regressed so that it became possible to perform a simple mastectomy. The combined endocrine and chemotherapy, thus, had achieved a 90% objective response rate in these patients. In a control group of patients selected randomly without HR assays, this modality of treatment only yielded a response rate less than 50%. One example of an HR-rich tumor can be illustrated by the following case history.

**Case No. B 81** — The female patient, aged 59, had a 7 × 6 × 4-cm-sized breast cancer wherein 90% of the cancer cells were positive for cytoplasmic estrogen and progesterone receptors. Enlarged lymph nodes were found in the axillary, supraclavicular, and cervical regions. As a case at the terminal stage ($T_4N_3M_1$), she was treated with a combination of tamoxifen and polychemotherapy. Two months later, the tumor size was reduced by 70%. A simple mastectomy and subsequent radiotherapy were performed. The administration of tamoxifen lasted 270 days. During the 25-month follow-up, she was in good condition without recurrence of new metastases.

## IV. DISCUSSION

The complex question of the mechanism of hormone secretion and its metabolism in subjects of high risk for breast cancer has so far not been well established. It has been the general belief that at least some breast cancers are intimately related to hormonal function and directly influenced by the level of estrogens in the blood. It is also known that steroid hormone receptors are present in the normal mammary glands which are capable of accepting hormonal stimuli with corresponding cellular response. During malignant transformation the receptor property of the cell may be partly or totally retained.[8-11]

Currently, there are several methods for evaluation of steroid hormone receptors in tissues; these include cytosol biochemical[12-14] and histochemical[15-18] assays. In the present study, we have adopted Lee's histochemical method for the assessment of hormone receptor-positive cancer cells in a series consisting of 145 patients with breast cancer, and the results of treatment are analyzed in relation to the hormone receptor status of the tumor with special reference to the use of this histochemical assay as a guidance in instituting combined endocrine and chemotherapeutic treatment. The relation of tumor receptor status to the histological type of the lesion, the menstrual status of the patient, the rate of survival, and the response to endocrine therapy as well as to nonendocrine treatment protocol are also explored.

Although many investigators have been successful in using histochemical techniques to detect estrogen and progesterone receptor-positive cancer cell, there has been practically no information available concerning the level of cancer cell receptor positivity that can be used as a threshold value to guide clinical treatment. Since most breast cancers are heterogeneous and are composed of receptor-positive and receptor-negative cells in varying proportions,[2] and since a minimum 50% reduction in tumor size has been generally accepted as an objective criterion for partial response to therapy, we have decided to use a 50% receptor-positive cancer cell population as a cutoff point. All breast cancers composed of 50% or a higher percentage of receptor-positive cancer cells are considered potentially responsive to endocrine manipulation. In practice, however, to determine accurately the percentage of receptor-positive cancer cells in a heterogeneous specimen which often contains several hundred thousand tumor cells dispersed among various noncancerous tissue structures is not an exact science and subject to human observation errors that could easily result in, say, a 10% deviation from the true number. This type of uncertainty is reflected in an artificially low number of cases allocated to the 40 to 49% cell-HR-positive group (Table 1); some tumors in this group have probably been placed by the examining pathologist into a higher or a lower category because of the implication in treatment involved. However, we do not consider this potential interpretative imprecision a serious drawback of the histochemical method, for any assay technique would place a certain number of cases in a "grey zone" around a cutoff point, finally calling for a human decision.

Our preliminary experience has confirmed that the cutoff point used to divide tumors into HR-rich and HR-poor groups as proposed is of practical value in predicting prognosis and in planning therapeutic protocols. As shown in Table 6, the survival rate of patients with advanced and terminal disease is significantly higher in the HR-rich group than in the poor group, irrespective of modalities of treatment. Thus, a patient presenting with an HR-rich breast cancer at terminal stage has a survival rate four times that expected for a patient with a HR-poor tumor.

When the objective criteria were applied to follow the late-stage pathologic lesions during treatment, 90% of the HR-rich tumors showed a complete or a partial response to the combined endocrine and chemotherapy, whereas less than 50% of the randomly selected tumors responded. This high response rate of 90% is probably induced by our combined endocrine and chemotherapy used to treat HR-rich breast cancers. The infiltrating cancer cell population in an HR-rich tumor is always heterogeneous. Chemotherapeutic agents are probably needed to inhibit the growth of the HR negative cancer cells of the tumor. The steroid receptor-poor cells may be, indeed, more sensitive to chemotherapeutic agents than the receptor-rich ones.[19]

When the primary and the secondary lesions were examined at the same time before systemic treatment was instituted, most breast cancers (72.7%) seemed to have an almost identical composition of receptor-positive and receptor-negative tumor cells in the primary lesion and the metastases. This is also consistent with the experience of others,[20,21] who have used cytosol biochemical assays to evaluate steroid receptor proteins. However, since breast cancer is known to be heterogeneous, it is not unexpected to find differences between the primary tumor and the metastatic lesions in the percentage of receptor-positive cancer cells during the course of the disease, especially under systemic treatment with chemotherapy and endocrine manipulation (Table 5).

It is well known that breast cancers of postmenopausal patients contain a higher concentration of estrogen receptor proteins than those tumors of premenopausal patients. Hawkins et al.[22] believed that during the menstruating age the low level of estrogen receptor proteins found in the tumor tissue homogenates is the result of a high rate of occupation of the binding sites by endogenous estrogens that are present in high concentrations in the peripheral blood. During the postmenopausal period, on the other hand, the blood level of endogenous estrogens is believed to be naturally lowered, while high levels of receptor proteins are maintained in the cytoplasm of the cancer cells. However, in MacDonald's report[23] of 23 postmenopausal women the estrogen level of the peripheral blood was found to reach a value two to five times that observed in premenopausal controls due to increased conversion of precursors. Thus, it appears that while the estrogen level is high in the menstruating age, it may become further elevated during the perimenopausal or postmenopausal period, a fact at variance with the postulation that the high hormone receptor protein assay value observed in the tumors during postmenopause is the results of decreased occupation by endogenous steroid hormones. Using ovariectomized adult female rats for study, Clark et al.[24] have shown that injection of estradiol increases the synthesis of estrogen receptors in the uterus whereas progesterone suppresses this effect. Therefore, if the hormone responsive cancers behave like an estrogen target organ, it seems possible that the high incidence of HR-rich breast cancers reported in the perimenopausal and postmenopausal period may be the result of an unopposed estrogenic stimulation on hormone responsive tumors due to cessation of production of progesterone by the ovaries.

In our series, the highest rate of HR-rich breast cancer is found in the subjects of the perimenopausal age group (62%), similar to that reported by Zhang,[25] whose data were based on biochemical cytosol assay of breast cancer among Chinese patients. However, when comparing the percentages between the HR-rich and the HR-poor tumors in the same age bracket (Table 2), there is no significant difference between the two, and the absolute number of cases may merely reflect the fact that breast cancer in Chinese women occurs mostly at an age when the effects of menopause begin to set in.

Among 141 female patients, 44% had HR-rich breast cancer. This percentage seems to be rather high. However, this is probably due to the fact that there is a high proportion of advanced cases among our patients. When the patients with early disease and the patients with advanced disease are considered separately, it becomes clear that the early cases have 28% of their tumors classified as HR-rich, similar to those reported by Lee.[2,26] The figure for advanced cases is about twice as high. It is not easy to explain why there is a disproportionately high incidence of HR-rich cancers in patients who presented with their disease at an advanced stage. One of the factors may be that the growth rate of these tumors tends to be slower so that the patients could tolerate the cancer for a longer period of time before seeking medical treatment.

McGuire et al.[10] reported that no correlation was found between the histological types of breast cancer and the levels of estrogen receptor proteins. However, a strong association between estrogen receptor level and infiltrating lobular carcinoma has been described,[27] although a later report from the same institution said that lobular carcinomas did not have a significantly higher incidence of estrogen receptor-positive tumors than ductal carcinomas.[28] In our series, mucinous carcinomas seem to have a tendency to contain a high percentage of receptor-positive cancer cells. Three papillary carcinomas and a case of Paget's disease have a low receptor status, with infiltrating ductal and infiltrating lobular carcinomas occupying an intermediate position. This experience is different from those of others who have reported papillary carcinomas[29] and Paget's disease[30] containing a significant number of receptor-positive cancer cells. We believe that no conclusion can be drawn on the relationship between steroid receptor status and the histological types of breast cancer at this time.

In summary, during a period of 3 years in which a fluorescent estrogen histochemical technique for steroid receptor assays was used to study breast cancers in our institution, we have accumulated both laboratory and clinical data to show that this histochemical approach is capable of identifying potentially hormone responsive breast cancers. The HR-rich cancers, as defined by our criteria, have a higher rate of response to endocrine therapy than the HR-poor tumors, and an HR-rich tumor generally indicates a longer survival rate for the patient. The value of this histochemical method in guiding clinical practice[31] is comparable to that achieved by the estrogen receptor protein assays as reported in the literature. The biological characteristics of the HR-rich and the HR-poor breast cancers as demonstrated in this series are similar to those of tumors with a high level of estrogen receptor proteins and with a low level of estrogen receptor proteins, respectively.

## REFERENCES

1. **Lee, S. H.,** Cytochemical study of estrogen receptor in human mammary cancer, *Am. J. Clin. Pathol.,* 70, 197, 1978.
2. **Lee, S. H.,** Cancer cell estrogen receptor of human mammary carcinoma, *Cancer,* 44, 1, 1979.
3. **Lee, S. H.,** Cellular estrogen and progesterone receptor in mammary carcinoma, *Am. J. Clin. Pathol.,* 73, 323, 1980.
4. **Lee, S. H.,** The histochemistry of estrogen receptors, *Histochemistry,* 71, 491, 1981.

5. **Yao, X., Meng, X., Chen, P., and Mei, Z.,** An assay of cellular sex steroid hormone receptors in mammary carcinoma, *Acta Acad. Med. Sichuan,* 13, 156, 1982.

6. **Chen, P., Mei, Z., Yao, X., and Meng, X.,** The significance for an assay of cellular sex steroid hormone receptor in the management of breast cancer, *Acta Acad. Med. Sichuan,* 13, 404, 1982.

7. **WHO,** The World Health Organization histological typing of breast tumors — second edition, *Am. J. Clin. Pathol.,* 78, 806, 1982.

8. **Folca, P. J., Glascock, R. F., and Irvin, W. T.,** Studies with tritium-labeled hexoestrol in advanced breast cancer, *Lancet,* 2, 796, 1961.

9. **Jensen, E. V., Block, G. E., Smith, S., Kyser, K., and DeSombre, E. R.,** Estrogen receptors and breast cancer response to adrenalectomy, *Natl. Cancer Inst. Monogr.,* 34, 55, 1971.

10. **McGuire, W. L., Carbone, P. P., Sears, M. E., and Escher, G. C.,** Estrogen receptors in human breast cancer, an overview, in *Estrogen Receptors in Human Breast Cancer,* McGuire, W. L., Carbone, P. P., and Vollmers, E. P., Eds., Raven Press, New York, 1975.

11. **McGuire, W. L., Horwitz, K. B., Pearson, O. H., and Segaloff, A.,** Current status of estrogen and progesterone receptors in breast cancer, *Cancer,* 39, 2934, 1977.

12. **Toft, D. O. and Gorski, J.,** A receptor molecule for estrogens: isolation from the rat uterus and preliminary characterization, *Proc. Natl. Acad. Sci. U.S.A.,* 55, 1574, 1966.

13. **Korenman, S. G.,** Radio-ligand binding assay of specific estrogens using a soluble uterine macromolecule, *J. Clin. Endocrinol. Metab.,* 28, 127, 1968.

14. **Garola, R. E. and McGuire, W. L.,** A hydroxyapatite micro-method for measuring estrogen receptor in human breast cancer, *Cancer Res.,* 38, 2216, 1978.

15. **Nenci, I., Beccati, M. D., Piffanelli, A., and Lanza, G.,** Detection and dynamic localization of estradiol-receptor complexes in intact target cells by immunofluorescence technique, *J. Steroid Biochem.,* 7, 505, 1976.

16. **Pertschuk, L. P.,** Detection of estrogen binding in human mammary carcinoma by immunofluorescence: a new technique utilizing the binding hormone in a polymerized state, *Res. Commun. Chem. Pathol. Pharmacol.,* 14, 771, 1976.

17. **Walker, R. A., Cove, D. H., and Howell, A.,** Histochemical detection of oestrogen receptor in human breast carcinomas, *Lancet,* 1, 171, 1980.

18. **Eusebi, V., Cerasoli, P. T., Guidelli-Guidi, S., Bussolati, G., and Azzopardi, J. G.,** A two-stage immunocytochemical method for oestrogen receptor analysis: correlation with morphological parameters of breast carcinomas, *Tumori,* 67, 315, 1981.

19. **Lippman, M. E., Allegra, J. C., Thompson, E. B., Simon, R., Barlock, A., Green, L., Huff, K. K., Do, H. M. T., Aitken, S. C., and Warren, R.,** The relation between estrogen receptors and response rate to cytotoxic chemotherapy in metastatic breast cancer, *N. Engl. J. Med.,* 298, 1223, 1978.

20. **Rosen, P. P., Menendez-Botet, C. J., Urban, J. A., Fracchia, A., and Schwartz, M. K.,** Estrogen receptor protein (ERP) in multiple tumor specimens from individual patients with breast cancer, *Cancer,* 39, 2194, 1977.

21. **Brennan, M. J., Donegan, W. L., and Appleby, D. E.,** The variability of estrogen receptors in metastatic breast cancer, *Am. J. Surg.,* 137, 260, 1979.

22. **Hawkins, R. A., Roberts, M. M., Freedman, B., Scott, K. M., Killen, E., and Forrest, A. P. M.,** Oestrogen receptors in human breast cancer: the Edinburgh experience, in *Steroid Receptor Assays in Human Breast Tumours: Methodological and Clinical Aspects,* King, R. J. B., Ed., Alpha Omega Publishing, Cardiff, 1979, chap. 4.

23. **Hemsell, D. L., Grodin, J. M., Brenner, P. F., Siiteri, P. K., and MacDonald, P. C.,** Plasma precursors of estrogen. II. Correlation of the extent of conversion of plasma androstenedione to estrone with age, *J. Clin. Endocrinol. Metab.,* 38, 476, 1974.

24. **Clark, J. H., Hsueh, A. J. W., and Peck, E. G., Jr.,** Regulation of estrogen receptor replenishment by progesterone, *Ann. N.Y. Acad. Sci.,* 286, 161, 1977.

25. **Zhang, H. Y.,** Steroid hormone receptor assay, Beijing Institute of Oncology, personal communication.

26. **Lee, S. H.,** Estrogen and progesterone receptors in breast cancer: a new approach to measure, *Conn. Med.,* 44, 622, 1980.

27. **Rosen, P. P., Menendez-Botet, C. J., Nisselbaum, J. S., Urban, J. A., Mike, V., Fracchia, A., and Schwartz, M. K.,** Pathological review of breast lesions analyzed for estrogen receptor protein, *Cancer Res.,* 35, 3187, 1975.

28. **Lesser, M. L., Rosen, P. P., Sennie, R. T., Duthie, K., Menendez-Botet, B., and Schwartz, M. K.,** Estrogen and progesterone receptors in breast carcinoma: correlations with epidemiology and pathology, *Cancer,* 48, 299, 1981.

29. **Lee, S. H.,** Sex steroid hormone receptors in mammary carcinoma, in *Diagnostic Immunohistochemistry,* DeLellis, R. A., Ed., Masson, New York, 1981, chap. 9.

30. **Fetissof, F., Lansac, J., and Arbeille-Brassart, B.,** Mise en évidence des récepteurs de l'oestradiol et de la progestérone sur preparations histologiques, *Ann. Anat. Pathol.,* 25, 201, 1980.
31. **Chen, P., Mei, Z., Yao, X., and Meng, X.,** Hormone receptor assessment for endocrine therapy in advanced breast cancer, *Chin. Med. J.,* 96, 751, 1983.

Chapter 5

# CANCER OF THE BREAST: CLINICOPATHOLOGICAL CORRELATIONS IN PRIMARY, RECURRENT, AND METASTATIC TUMORS WITH HISTOCHEMICALLY DETERMINED HORMONE RECEPTORS

**Pietro Lampertico and Franca Stagni**

## TABLE OF CONTENTS

I.    Introduction ................................................................. 64

II.   Methods and Materials ....................................................... 66

III.  Results ..................................................................... 67
      A.    Age Distribution ...................................................... 67
      B.    Tumor Size ............................................................ 67
      C.    Lymph Node Involvement ................................................ 68
      D.    Pathological Staging .................................................. 70
      E.    Tumor Margin .......................................................... 71
      F.    Multicentricity ....................................................... 72
      G.    Histotype ............................................................. 72
      H.    Vascular Invasion ..................................................... 75

IV.   Clinical Course ............................................................. 75

V.    Conclusions ................................................................. 80

Acknowledgments ................................................................. 81

References ...................................................................... 81

## I. INTRODUCTION

At the hospital of Busto Arsizio, a town of 80,000 inhabitants, in the Province of Varese, Lombardy, 1741 invasive breast cancers were histologically documented between 1950 and 1979. In Busto Arsizio, the incidence of breast cancer increased from 34.6/100,000 women in 1950 to 1954 to 76.1/100,000 women in 1975 to 1979.[1] The high incidence of breast carcinoma in this region has been previously noted in a study of tumor mortality by Cislaghi et al.[2] as well as by the Registro Tumori della Lombardia.[3] Between 1976 and 1977, 648 cases were discovered in the Province of Varese for an incidence of 80.7/100,000 women.[3]

In our institution, patients with breast cancer have been treated by conventional means and, more recently, according to the Foncam protocols.[4] However, there are no facilities for the biochemical measurement of steroid hormone receptors. Following reports detailing the histochemical demonstration of steroid hormone binding sites $(R_f)$,[5-7] we systematically applied the method of Lee to the majority of primary and recurrent breast tumors from October 1980 to the present.

The need for a simple method for performing steroid binding analyses was emphasized at an informal meeting held in Milan in April 1983[8] at which 13 different laboratory groups reported their results on more than 1300 determinations made by the Lee procedure. It was agreed by all participants that the methodology was simple. Gambacorta[9] discussed a method for the hematoxylin staining of the same sections employed for histochemistry, which allowed for a detailed morphological study of positive and negative cells and for their distribution. Lunetta[10] emphasized the importance of selecting multiple areas from larger tumors, especially from the periphery. Stagni et al.[11] showed their application of the histochemical method to cytological material obtained either by scraping the cut surface of a neoplasm or by thin-needle aspiration. Slides were kept at $-25°C$ for 10 to 15 min and then processed. Scrapings resulted in a richly cellular smear which permitted an easy and more accurate appraisal of negative and positive cells as well as an evaluation of their staining intensity. These workers emphasized that the strong fluorescence observed in cell clumps should best be avoided and evaluations be limited to single cells. They believed that scraping should be complementary to tissue section study and not an alternative. However, the analysis of material obtained by thin-needle aspiration might occasionally be the only method applicable to advanced cases of breast cancer. In some instances, as reported by Pertschuk,[12] malignant pleural effusions may also be studied in a similar manner.

The majority of investigators at the Milan meeting used normal mammary tissue or fibroadenoma as positive substrate controls and nontarget tissue as negative substrate controls. Antoci et al.[13] preincubated tissue sections with unconjugated estrogens and obtained inhibition of ligand binding. On selected cases, the same group attempted semiquantification of positive tumors by limiting dilution studies, as suggested by Meijer et al.,[14] and obtained satisfactory correlations with biochemical assays. A simple method of photometric evaluation might be obtained by studying the exposure time required for photography, or fluorescence quenching. A more sophisticated and precise approach using computer-assisted microfluorometry was reported by Pertschuk.[15] Computerized morphometric analysis was also employed by Gambacorta[16] in order to more precisely determine the distribution of cancer cells and stroma.

Some heterogeneity was apparent in the results obtained by the various participants at the Milan conference. A possible reason was because in some institutions all accessioned specimens were studied, while in others histochemistry was only performed upon request of the clinician. Overall, 64% of 1300 histochemical estrogen binding assays were positive $(R_f +)$ or borderline. Six of the laboratories reporting had a deviation from this value $\pm$ 10. In others, the deviation was higher. In three laboratories, each with over 150 assays, the

**Table 1**

**HISTOCHEMICAL ASSAYS FROM 13
ITALIAN LABORATORIES**

| Laboratory | No. of cases | $R_f+$ (%) | Deviation from average |
|---|---|---|---|
| 1 | 302 | 54 | −10 |
| 2 | 217 | 55 | −9 |
| 3 | 176 | 53 | −11 |
| 4 | 86 | 92 | +28 |
| 5 | 69 | 96 | +32 |
| 6 | 69 | 45 | −19 |
| 7 | 60 | 55 | −9 |
| 8 | 60 | 64 | ±0 |
| 9 | 50 | 42 | −22 |
| 10 | 39 | 94 | +30 |
| 11 | 38 | 55 | −9 |
| 12 | 36 | 74 | +10 |
| 13 | 20 | 45 | −19 |
| Total | 1.264 | Av 64% | |

**Table 2**

**ER[a] DISTRIBUTION IN BIOCHEMICALLY
ASSAYED CANCERS**

| No. of cases | ER+ (%) | Deviation from average | Ref. |
|---|---|---|---|
| 748 | 51 | −9.6 | 17 |
| 735 | 72 | +11.4 | 18 |
| 421 | 77 | +16.4 | 19 |
| 398 | 45.2 | −15.4 | 20 |
| 324 | 58 | −2.6 | 21 |
| 178 | 47.8 | −12.8 | 22 |
| 140 | 73 | +12.4 | 23 |
| Total 2.980 | Av 60.6% | | |

[a]  ER = estrogen receptor.

percentage of positive cases was surprisingly close (Table 1). This close relationship was statistically significant by the Fisher test and was suggestive of a high degree of reproducibility of assay results in these three institutions, each with a large number of unselected cases. A brief literature review revealed that similar wide excursions of positivity have been previously reported for biochemical assays (Table 2), with the average number of positive specimens being 61%.[17-23] The average positivity in a smaller series of specimens studied by histochemistry was 63% (Table 3 — top half), with a less-marked deviation from the average than in the current series.[7,24-27] Table 3 — bottom half — shows a small series of cases studied by immunohistochemical methods with even more consistent results.[27-29] It, thus, appears that histochemical and biochemical assays gave similar average percentages of positivity between 60 and 64% while for immunohistochemistry, this value was 71%. Variance analyses by both the Fischer and Student tests showed that the median values by all three methods did not differ significantly.

**Table 3**
## $R_f+$ DISTRIBUTION IN
## MORPHOLOGICALLY ASSAYED CANCERS

| | No. of cases | $R_f+$ (%) | Deviation from average | Ref. |
|---|---|---|---|---|
| | 363 | 62 | −0.8 | 24 |
| | 52 | 52 | −10.8 | 7 |
| | 48 | 62.5 | −0.3 | 25 |
| | 46 | 69.9 | +7.1 | 26 |
| | 26 | 85 | +23.8 | 27 |
| Total | 535 | Av 62.8% | | |
| | 277 | 71.1 | −0.3 | 28 |
| | 26 | 77 | +6.6 | 27 |
| | 12 | 75 | +3.6 | 29 |
| Total | 315 | Av 71.4% | | |

Following the Milan meeting, the Italian Society of Hospital Pathologists decided to pursue these studies, in particular, in order to determine the relationship between steroid binding as determined by the method of Lee, prognosis, and response to endocrine manipulation. Although much basic information has been published concerning assays of this type,[30-34] the clinicopathologic correlations remain scant,[25-27,35,36] primarily because insufficient time has elapsed since the advent of these procedures.

In this chapter we will review in detail our own experience with the Lee technique, particularly its relationship to anatomopathological features and, in a few instances, with clinical behavior and response to therapy.

## II. METHODS AND MATERIALS

Between October 1980 and August 1983 histochemical steroid binding assays were performed on 356 primary breast tumors primarily removed in our own hospital, although a few specimens excised at other institutions were also studied. The assay was also performed on several local cutaneous recurrences and occasional distant metastases. In 24 inoperable primary or metastatic lesions material obtained by fine-needle aspiration was studied. Positive and negative substrate controls included endometrium, myometrium, and intestine. Several specimens of kidney and renal cell carcinoma were also studied.[37]

Specimens sent to the laboratory for frozen section diagnosis were rapidly frozen in $CO_2$ and extra sections cut for histochemistry. Mastectomy specimens were dissected, usually within 2 hr of removal, and the tumor isolated. When the tumor was small the sample studied was representative of the entire lesion. When larger tumors were encountered a specimen from the infiltrating margin was taken. The only modification to the method described by Lee[7] was the study of smears derived by scraping the cut surface of the tumors. These smears as well as fine-needle aspirates were placed in a freezer for 10 to 15 min and then processed exactly as were the tumor sections. The single estrogen or progesterone ligand, or the combined reagent (Fluoro-cep®, Zeus Scientific, Raritan, N. J.) were employed. Processed sections were studied with a Leitz Orthomat microscope using reflected UV light by at least two observers. When strong fluorescence was observed in >50% of the observed tumor cells the case was assigned into the $R_f+$ category. Initially, cases exhibiting strong fluorescence in 30 to 50% of the cancer cells were considered to be borderline positive. However, we currently include such cases in the $R_f+$ group. When the tissue sections were unsatisfactory because of artifact, or a clear determination as to positivity or negativity was in doubt, then the parallel smear was examined. At least 500 tumor cells were inspected and differentiated into positive or negative groups. The degree of fluorescent intensity was also ascertained. Histochemical assays were usually processed and read the day of surgery. Identical techniques were used for estrogen and progesterone.

All cases were classified as to pathological TNM categories and by histologic diagnoses. Clinical data were gathered from each patient's chart. Follow-up data were gathered from the files of the breast cancer outpatient department and radiology department. Data processing and analyses were performed at the Centro di Calcolo Elettronico dell 'Università Cattolica in Busto Arsizio. The chi square test was used for statistical analyses; $p$ values $<0.05$ were considered significant.

We considered the following clinical and histologic parameters in relation to steroid binding: (1) age distribution, (2) tumor size (T), (3) lymph node involvement (N), (4) pathological staging, (5) tumor margin, (6) multicentricity, (7) histotype, (8) vascular invasion, and, where possible, (9) clinical course of disease.

## III. RESULTS

Of the 356 primary tumors studied, 204 (57.3%) were positive and 152 (42.7%) negative. No significant differences were noted between estrogen and progesterone binding assays.

### A. Age Distribution

Patients with primary breast cancers were stratified in two ways: (1) as premenopausal (<44 years), perimenopausal (45 to 54 years), and postmenopausal (>55 years); and (2) by 5-year periods (Figure 1).

Table 4 shows the distribution of $R_f+$ and $R_f-$ cases by 5-year periods. Negative cases prevailed prior to age 44 with a peak of increased positivity between ages 45 and 49 years. With the exception of the next 5-year period, in older women positive cases outnumbered the negative cases. Comparison of the distribution of cases showed that positive cases increased by age until 49 years. There was then an abrupt decrease in women ages 50 to 54. Thereafter, there was a constant relationship between $R_f+$ cases and age. On the other hand, except for women between 50 and 54 years, the number of negative cases increased with decreasing age. It is possible that the findings in the 50- to 54-year-old group of patients were related to hormonal imbalance during this stage of life. Indeed, the greatest percentage of negative cases occurred in this group. Elwood and Godolphin[18] divided 735 cases of breast cancer by 5-year periods and showed similar results including the 50-to 54-year old group. The latter observation by both histochemistry and biochemistry may be of considerable importance and worthy of verification. Most workers who merely subdivide their cases into pre-, peri-, and postmenopausal categories would fail to notice this strange distribution between ages 50 and 54.[17,22,23,25,26]

### B. Tumor Size

Tumors with a diameter under 2.0 cm (T1) constituted 52% of the group studied. Table 5 shows that this was the largest group, with tumors ranging in size from 2.0 to 5.0 cm (T2) constituting the second largest. Tumors larger than 5.0 cm were uncommon. Prior epidemiological investigations of this locale in Italy showed that between 1950 and 1979, tumors <2.0 cm represented only 13% of the total in the first decade, whereas this increased to 42.8% in the third decade.[1] Between 1980 and 1983 there was a further increase in early diagnosis of breast cancers with the percentage of small tumors becoming progressively greater. This fact is of great importance for histochemical steroid binding assays which require very much less tissue than biochemical methods.

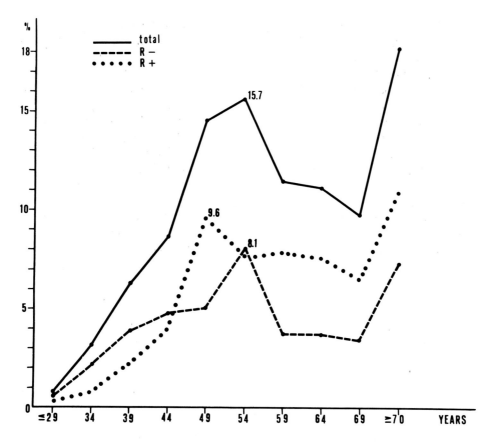

FIGURE 1.   Percentage 5-year distribution of 356 primary breast cancers and subdivision according to $R_f$ (fluorescent steroid binding) status.

In the T1 tumors there were more $R_f+$ than $R_f-$ specimens (65.4% vs. 34.6% of 185 cancers). Of 142 T2 tumors, there was a slight prevalence in the number of $R_f-$ specimens (51.4% vs. 48.6%). In the small number of T3 and T4 cancers there were no significant differences between the percentage of positive and negative specimens.

A more accurate analysis of steroid binding and tumor size was attempted according to menopausal status. In patients <44 years of age there was an equal distribution of positive and negative cases in the T1 category, while $R_f-$ cases predominated in the T2 group. In the perimenopausal patients, the T1 lesions were primarily $R_f+$, while the T2, T3, and T4 tumors were mainly $R_f-$ (Figures 2A and 2B). $R_f+$ cases predominated in the older women (Figure 2C). The different distribution in the perimenopausal women was statistically significant ($p = 0.0104$). A significant relationship between tumor size and receptor status was not found by other workers.[23,38]

## C. Lymph Node Involvement

Histological examination of lymph nodes was performed in 338 cases. Table 6 shows that 183 (54.1%) had no nodal involvement (NO) while 155 (45.9%) had nodal metastases (N1 or N2). No significant differences were apparent in $R_f$ either in the group as a whole or by age subgroup. Others[38,39] have reported similar findings with biochemical receptor data.

**Table 4**
**STRATIFICATION OF $R_f$ BY 5-YEAR PERIODS**

| | ≤29 | 30—34 | 35—39 | 40—44 | 45—49 | 50—54 | 55—59 | 60—64 | 65—69 | ≥70 | Total |
|---|---|---|---|---|---|---|---|---|---|---|---|
| No. $R_f$− | 2 | 8 | 14 | 17 | 18 | 29 | 13 | 13 | 12 | 26 | 152 |
| $R_f$− cases (%) | 1.3 | 5.3 | 9.2 | 11.2 | 11.8 | 19.1 | 8.6 | 8.6 | 7.9 | 17.1 | |
| Age group (%) | 66.7 | 72.7 | 63.6 | 54.8 | 34.6 | 51.8 | 31.7 | 32.5 | 34.3 | 40 | |
| Total % | 0.6 | 2.2 | 3.9 | 4.8 | 5.1 | 8.1 | 3.7 | 3.7 | 3.4 | 7.3 | 42.7 |
| | | | | | | | | | | | |
| No. $R_f$+ | 1 | 3 | 8 | 14 | 34 | 27 | 28 | 27 | 23 | 39 | 204 |
| $R_f$+ cases (%) | 0.5 | 1.5 | 3.9 | 6.9 | 16.7 | 13.2 | 13.7 | 13.2 | 11.3 | 19.1 | |
| Age group (%) | 33.3 | 27.3 | 36.4 | 45.2 | 65.4 | 48.2 | 68.3 | 67.5 | 65.7 | 60 | |
| Total (%) | 0.3 | 0.8 | 2.2 | 3.9 | 9.6 | 7.6 | 7.9 | 7.6 | 6.5 | 11 | 57.3 |
| | | | | | | | | | | | |
| Total no. | 3 | 11 | 22 | 31 | 52 | 56 | 41 | 40 | 35 | 65 | 356 |
| Age group (%) | 0.8 | 3.1 | 6.2 | 8.7 | 14.6 | 15.7 | 11.5 | 11.2 | 9.8 | 18.3 | 100 |

*Note:* Chi square = 18.77727, $p$ = 0.0272.

**Table 5**
**R$_f$ AND TUMOR SIZE**

|  | T1 | T2 | T3 | T4 | Total |
|---|---|---|---|---|---|
| No. R$_f$− | 64 | 73 | 6 | 9 | 152 |
| R$_f$− cases (%) | 42.1 | 48 | 3.9 | 5.9 | |
| T (%) | 34.6 | 51.4 | 50 | 52.9 | |
| Total (%) | 18 | 20.5 | 1.7 | 2.5 | 42.7 |
| | | | | | |
| No. R$_f$+ | 121 | 69 | 6 | 8 | 204 |
| R$_f$+ cases (%) | 59.3 | 33.8 | 2.9 | 3.9 | |
| T (%) | 65.4 | 48.6 | 50 | 47.1 | |
| Total (%) | 34 | 19.4 | 1.7 | 2.2 | 57.3 |
| | | | | | |
| Total no. | 185 | 142 | 12 | 17 | 356 |
| Total T (%) | 52 | 39.9 | 3.4 | 4.8 | 100 |

*Note:* Chi square $= 10.35917$, $p = 0.0157$.

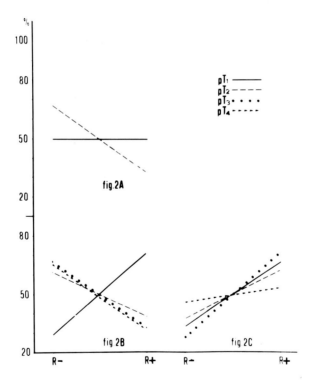

FIGURE 2.   Tumor size (T) and R$_f$ distribution in patients below age 44 (Figure 2A), between 45 and 54 (Figure 2B), and over age 55 (Figure 2C).

## D. Pathological Staging

Staging of disease, by evaluation of the various features of a tumor including possible extension to axillary lymph nodes as recommended by the UICC,[40] is considered of more prognostic significance than tumor size or lymph node involvement alone and is a guide to therapeutic procedures. We have divided our cases into the various pathological stages in relation to their histochemical steroid binding data.

**Table 6**
**R$_f$ AND AXILLARY LYMPH NODE**
**INVOLVEMENT**

|  | N0 | N1 | N2 | Total |
|---|---|---|---|---|
| No. R$_f$– | 76 | 63 | 7 | 146 |
| R$_f$– cases (%) | 52.1 | 43.2 | 4.8 | |
| In category (%) | 41.5 | 44.1 | 58.3 | |
| Total (%) | 22.5 | 18.6 | 2.1 | 43.2 |
| | | | | |
| No. R$_f$+ | 107 | 80 | 5 | 192 |
| R$_f$+ cases (%) | 55.7 | 41.7 | 2.6 | |
| In category (%) | 58.5 | 55.9 | 41.7 | |
| Total (%) | 31.7 | 23.7 | 1.5 | 56.8 |
| | | | | |
| Total no. | 183 | 143 | 12 | 338 |
| In category (%) | 54.1 | 42.3 | 3.6 | 100 |

*Note:* Chi square = 1.37071, $p$ = 0.5039.

Patients with primary tumors considered to be R$_f$+ represented the majority (68.5%) of those classified into stage 1, about one half of the stage 2 patients, and less than half of the stages 3a and 3b cases. The percentage of positive specimens again increased in stage 4 (Table 7).

In Figure 3, staging and R$_f$ are related to the three age groups. In stage 1 R$_f$+ cases were prevalent in all age groups, especially in perimenopausal women. On the contrary, in stage 2, women below age 54 were mostly R$_f$– ($p$ = 0.0004). In stage 3a, five women under age 44 were R$_f$–, in four patients 45 to 54 years old there was an equal distribution of R$_f$+ and R$_f$–, while ten older women were mostly positive (70%; $p$ = 0.0375). In stage 3b the difference in distribution was not significant. In stage 4, there were only eight patients, five R$_f$+ and three R$_f$–.

Comparison of the R$_f$ status of tumors classified as stage 1 and 2 (Figure 3A and B) with those defined only by size (T1 and T2; Figures 2A, B, and C) shows that graphs of stage 2 and T2 are not significantly different, while a remarkable difference is present in stage 1 patients under age 44 who were much more likely to be R$_f$+. The reason for this difference is shown in Table 8. It is apparent that R$_f$– cases under age 54 more commonly had lymph node metastases than R$_f$+ cases. However, chi square analyses of these data were not significant ($p$ >0.05).

**E. Tumor Margin**

A circumscribed tumor margin may be suggestive of less aggressive behavior than a margin which is irregular and extends into the adjacent fat. In our material observations as to tumor margins were made by both gross and microscopic examination in 342 cases. Only 53 were considered to be well circumscribed. It is possible that the margin determination as to circumscription was underestimated in the current series. In a series of cases evaluated by Fisher,[40] the percentage distribution was 39.8% of gross vs. 16.9% microscopic circumscription. Table 9 shows that division of the specimens according to R$_f$ revealed that tumors with a more rounded margin were more often R$_f$– (66%), while 61.9% of R$_f$+ lesions had an irregular margin. Although no such relationships have been described by others,[38,39] our results are statistically significant ($p$ = 0.0003).

**Table 7**
**$R_f$ AND PATHOLOGICAL STAGE**

|  | $R_f$-negative | $R_f$-positive | Total |
|---|---|---|---|
| Stage X |  |  |  |
| No. | 4 | 8 | 12 |
| In stage (%) | 33.6 | 66.7 |  |
| $R_f$ (%) | 2.6 | 3.9 |  |
| Total (%) | 1.1 | 2.2 | 3.4 |
| Stage 1 |  |  |  |
| No. | 39 | 85 | 124 |
| In stage (%) | 31.5 | 68.5 |  |
| $R_f$ (%) | 25.7 | 41.6 |  |
| Total (%) | 11 | 23.9 | 34.8 |
| Stage 2 |  |  |  |
| No. | 89 | 92 | 181 |
| In stage (%) | 49.2 | 50.9 |  |
| $R_f$ (%) | 58.6 | 45.1 |  |
| Total (%) | 25 | 25.9 | 50.8 |
| Stage 3a |  |  |  |
| No. | 10 | 9 | 19 |
| In stage (%) | 52.6 | 47.4 |  |
| $R_f$ (%) | 6.6 | 4.4 |  |
| Total (%) | 2.8 | 2.5 | 5.3 |
| Stage 3b |  |  |  |
| No. | 7 | 5 | 12 |
| In stage (%) | 58.3 | 41.6 |  |
| $R_f$ (%) | 4.6 | 2.5 |  |
| Total (%) | 2 | 1.4 | 3.4 |
| Stage 4 |  |  |  |
| No. | 3 | 5 | 8 |
| In stage (%) | 37.5 | 62.5 |  |
| $R_f$ (%) | 2 | 2.5 |  |
| Total (%) | 0.8 | 1.4 | 2.2 |
|  |  |  |  |
| Total no. | 152 | 204 | 356 |
| $R_f$ (%) | 42.7 | 57.3 | 100 |

*Note:* Chi square = 11.99393, $p < 0.05$.

## F. Multicentricity

Gross and/or microscopic examination revealed multiple nodules within the same breast in 45 cases (12.1%). In 15 cases multiple histochemical assays were performed (one per nodule). Only in two instances were assays of multiple nodules at variance and, in most instances, there was no difference in results between one and another nodule within the same breast. There was a slight preponderance of $R_f-$ cases in this group (Table 10) but this was not statistically significant ($p > 0.05$). Hull et al.,[42] reporting on 54 simultaneous assays of eight cases with multiple primary tumors, found only one instance of discordance.

## G. Histotype

Table 11 shows the steroid binding distribution in relation to the histopathological diagnosis. High rates of positivity were observed in tubular (100%) and colloid (71.4%) carcinomas; 68% of lobular and 56.8% of ductal carcinomas were also positive. Medullary and anaplastic tumors were usually negative. Positivity in lobular carcinomas was higher in perimenopausal women (72.7%) and constant in the other age groups (66.7%). In ductal carcinomas, positivity increased by age almost approaching the percentage of the lobular

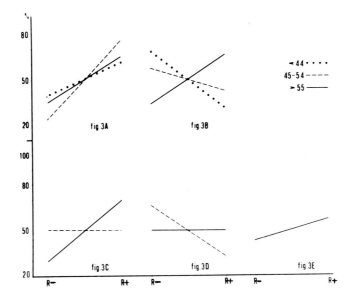

FIGURE 3.   Age groupings and $R_f$ distribution in stage 1 (Figure 3A), stage 2 (Figure 3B), stage 3a (Figure 3C), stage 3b (Figure 3D), and in stage 4 (Figure 3E).

**Table 8**
**$R_f$ DISTRIBUTION OF T1 TUMORS IN STAGE 1 CASES AND IN MORE ADVANCED STAGES**

| Ages (years) | $R_f$ | T1 no. of cases | Stage 1 No. | % | More advanced stages No. | % |
|---|---|---|---|---|---|---|
| ≤44 | – | 15 | 7 | 47 | 8 | 53 |
| | + | 15 | 11 | 73 | 4 | 27 |
| | | Chi square 1.25 | | | $p>0.05$ | |
| 45—54 | – | 18 | 10 | 55 | 8 | 45 |
| | + | 43 | 33 | 77 | 10 | 23 |
| | | Chi square 1.814723 | | | $p>0.05$ | |
| ≥55 | – | 31 | 22 | 71 | 9 | 29 |
| | + | 63 | 41 | 65 | 22 | 35 |
| | | Chi square 0.1139569 | | | $p>0.05$ | |
| Total | | 185 | 124 | 67 | 61 | 33 |
| | | Chi square 1.247572 | | | $p>0.05$ | |

type in older women (35.4:54.4:66.4% for the pre-, peri-, and postmenopausal groups; Figure 4). This difference was highly significant ($p = 0.001$).

In the series of 2980 breast cancers assayed biochemically and collected by Underwood,[43] ductal carcinomas had a median positivity of 62% (range: 46 to 77%) and lobular carcinomas 80% (range: 49 to 100%). Medullary carcinomas had a mean positivity of 26% (range: 9 to 58%). Thus, there were no significant differences as to positivity between histochemical and biochemical assay results in the more common breast tumors. The relatively uncommon tubular carcinoma was consistently more positive in the current series, while biochemical

### Table 9
### $R_f$ AND TUMOR MARGIN

| Type of margin | $R_f$-positive | $R_f$-negative | Total |
|---|---|---|---|
| Regular | | | |
| No. | 18 | 35 | 53 |
| Regular (%) | 34 | 66 | |
| $R_f$ (%) | 9.1 | 24.1 | |
| Total (%) | 5.3 | 10.2 | 15.5 |
| Irregular | | | |
| No. | 179 | 110 | 289 |
| Irregular (%) | 61.9 | 38.1 | |
| $R_f$ (%) | 90.9 | 75.9 | |
| Total (%) | 52.3 | 32.2 | 84.5 |
| | | | |
| Total no. | 197 | 145 | 342 |
| $R_f$ (%) | 57.6 | 42.5 | 100 |

*Note:* Chi square = 13.22960, $p$ = 0.0003.

### Table 10
### $R_f$ AND MULTICENTRIC TUMORS

| | No. of cases | $R_f +$ | | $R_f -$ | |
|---|---|---|---|---|---|
| | | No. | % | No. | % |
| Single tumors | 313 | 182 | 58.1 | 131 | 41.9 |
| Multicentric tumors | 43 | 22 | 51.2 | 21 | 48.8 |
| | | | | | |
| Total | 356 | 204 | 57.5 | 152 | 42.5 |

*Note:* Chi square = 0.4953054, $p$ > 0.05.

### Table 11
### $R_f$ AND HISTOPATHOLOGIC DIAGNOSES

| Histotypes | Total no. of cases | % | $R_f +$ | | $R_f -$ | |
|---|---|---|---|---|---|---|
| | | | No. | % | No. | % |
| Ductal | 252 | 70.8 | 143 | 56.8 | 109 | 43.2 |
| Lobular | 47 | 13.2 | 32 | 68.1 | 15 | 31.9 |
| Medullary | 13 | 3.7 | 3 | 23.1 | 10 | 76.9 |
| Tubular | 6 | 1.6 | 6 | 100.0 | | |
| Gelatinous | 7 | 2.0 | 5 | 71.4 | 2 | 28.6 |
| Mixed | 16 | 4.4 | 10 | 62.5 | 6 | 37.5 |
| Anaplastic | 4 | 1.1 | | | 4 | 100.0 |
| Apocrine | 2 | 0.6 | 1 | 50.0 | 1 | 50.0 |
| Papillary | 2 | 0.6 | 1 | 50.0 | 1 | 50.0 |
| Intraductal | 5 | 1.4 | 3 | 60.0 | 2 | 40.0 |
| Others | 2 | 0.6 | | | 2 | 100.0 |
| | | | | | | |
| Total | 356 | 100.0 | 204 | 57.3 | 152 | 42.7 |

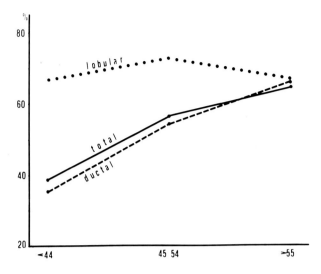

FIGURE 4.   Distribution of $R_f$ positivity in three main age groups for the entire series and for ductal and lobular carcinomas.

assay results were more variable.[43] Some observers have related high positivity in this tumor to its relatively advanced state of differentiation.[35] Parl and Wagner[23] reported positivity in 95% of highly differentiated tumors and 79 and 64%, respectively, in those of medium and low grades of differentiation. A similar relationship, also reported by others,[44,45] was not sought for in this study.

## H. Vascular Invasion

Cancer cells in vascular channels were present in 76 specimens. Forty-six were in $R_f +$ tumors and 35 in $R_f -$ lesions. This finding, similar to that reported earlier,[38] was not significant.

## IV. CLINICAL COURSE

Only a brief period of time has elapsed since the initial application of the histochemical method in our laboratory. In the last months of 1980, 19 assays were performed. In 1981, 151 and in 1982, 131 determinations were made. In addition, 87 were performed in 1983 to the present time.

We have reviewed clinical data, including previously reported material[46] to August 1983; 54% of patients had one or more clinical follow-up visits after initial surgery, especially patients with $R_f -$ tumors (Table 12). Progression of disease was noted in 45 patients representing 15 and 29% of the $R_f +$ and $R_f -$ cases, respectively. This was a statistically significant difference ($p < 0.05$). Death occurred in nine patients (2.6% of $R_f +$, 6.25% of $R_f -$ groups). Even in stage 1, progression of disease was more noticeable in $R_f -$ cases, but this was not statistically significant.

Cutaneous recurrences occurred in 11 patients, were evaluated histochemically and/or cytochemically, and the results compared with those of initial assay of the primary tumor. Cutaneous recurrences were also studied in 19 other women who underwent mastectomy prior to 1980, or were originally operated on in other hospitals. No major discordances were noted between the primary and recurrence assay results in the 11 cases, although different degrees of positivity were apparent. Twenty-five of the latter 30 patients had an excision of their recurrence, while in 5, fine-needle aspirations were performed. The time prior to tumor

**Table 12**
**EVOLUTION OF DISEASE IN PATIENTS WITH KNOWN $R_f$**

| $R_f$ | Stage | Total no. of cases | No. with follow-up | Progression of disease No. | Progression of disease % | Died |
|---|---|---|---|---|---|---|
| Positive | 1 | 85 | 44 | 6 | 13.6 | 1 |
| | 2 | 92 | 52 | 7 | 13.4 | |
| | 3a | 9 | 7 | 2 | 28.6 | |
| | 3b | 5 | 0 | | | |
| | 4 | 5 | 2 | 2 | 100 | 2 |
| | X | 8 | 4 | 0 | | |
| | Secondary tumors | 21 | 4 | 0 | | |
| | Total | 225 | 113 | 17 | 15 | 3 |
| Negative | 1 | 39 | 14 | 4 | 28.5 | |
| | 2 | 89 | 64 | 14 | 21.8 | 4 |
| | 3a | 10 | 7 | 3 | 42.8 | 1 |
| | 3b | 7 | 6 | 3 | 50 | |
| | 4 | 3 | 2 | 2 | 66.6 | |
| | X | 4 | 0 | | | |
| | Secondary tumors | 11 | 3 | 2 | 66.6 | 1 |
| | Total | 163 | 96 | 28 | 29 | 6 |

recurrence was longer in those patients with $R_f+$ tumors (average 55.5 months) than in those with $R_f-$ cancers (21.8 months; Table 13).

In a large series of sequential pairs of assays from 161 patients studied biochemically, Hull et al.[42] found major discordances between the initial and subsequent assays. However, some patients had been subjected to endocrine manipulation in the interim. Harland et al.[47] found a 23% variation in estrogen receptor and a 30% variation in progesterone receptor assays in 88 double determinations. Both authors analyzed, in depth, possible reasons for these discrepancies. Heterogeneity of the samples analyzed as well as the possibility of errors in measurement were thought to be responsible.

In our group of 30 patients with recurrent or metastatic diseases (Table 14), $R_f-$ cases predominated (60%), whereas such tumors comprised only 42.7% of all of the primary tumors examined. Table 15 relates the disease-free interval and staging to $R_f$. The disease-free interval was shorter in negative cases in stages 2, 3a, and, in particular, stage 4. Roberts and Hannel[38] noticed a slightly longer disease-free interval between biochemically positive and negative cases (16.5 months vs. 8.6 months). Similar results were reported by Crowe et al.[48] in stage 1, postmenopausal women, by Heise and Gorlish[49] and by Kinne et al.[50]

The results of postmastectomy therapy have been subjected to preliminary analysis in two groups of patients: (1) in a group of women given adjuvant therapy and (2) in all patients receiving endocrine therapy. Seven patients in the first group who were $R_f+$ received some form of endocrine therapy alone or in combination. None showed disease progression. Five patients were $R_f-$, three of whom evidenced progression of disease. No significant differences were noted between $R_f+$ and $R_f-$ patients treated with nonhormonal modalities (Table 16). These results with adjuvant endocrine therapy in $R_f+$ cases suggest good specificity and sensitivity for histochemistry. However, too few cases have been studied for the findings to be statistically significant. In the group of patients who received nonhormonal adjuvant therapy, progression of disease in positive and negative cases occurred at approximately the same rate. Similar findings have been reported by Kinne et al.[50]

## Table 13
## $R_f$ IN CUTANEOUS RECURRENCES

| TN | No. of cases | $R_f$ in PT | Status in CR | Age Median | Age Range | Free interval Median | Free interval Range |
|---|---|---|---|---|---|---|---|
| T1 N0 | 3 | + in 2 u. in 1 | + | 62 | 54—76 | 51 | 21—60 |
|  | 3 | − in 1 u. in 2 | − | 46 | 29—58 | 35 | 13—72 |
| T1 N1b | 4 | + in 1 u. in 3 | + | 57 | 49—63 | 25 | 11—36 |
|  | 3 | − in 3 | − | 49 | 29—65 | 14 | 12—15 |
| T2 N0 | 3 | + in 1 u. in 2 | + | 70 | 57—77 | 103 | 22—180 |
|  | 2 | − in 1 u. in 1 | − | 50 | 36—64 | 48 | 16—33 |
| T2 N1 | 2 | u. in 2 | + (1 c) | 57 | 55—59 | 35 | 23—48 |
| T3 | 1 | u. | + (1 c) | 42 | 42 | 9 | 9 |
|  | 1 | u. | − | 81 | 81 | 7 | 7 |
| T4b | 2 | − in 2 | − | 75 | 73—77 | 3 | 3 |
| Tx Nx | 2 | u. | + (1 c) | 60 | 52—67 | 96 | 84—102 |
|  | 4 | u. | − (2 c) | 69 | 64—78 | 18 (u. in 1) | 9—36 |

*Note:* PT = primary tumor; CR = cutaneous recurrence; u. = unknown; c = assay performed on cytological material.

## Table 14
## METASTASES IN PATIENTS
## WITH KNOWN $R_f$

| Metastatic sites | No. of cases | Receptor status $R_f+$ | Receptor status $R_f-$ |
|---|---|---|---|
| Multiple | 9 | 1 | 8 |
| Lymphnodes | 7 | 2 | 5 |
| Bones | 7 | 4 | 3 |
| Lungs | 4 | 3 | 1 |
| Liver | 1 | 1 | — |
| Serous cavities | 1 | 1 | — |
| Brain | 1 | — | 1 |
| Total | 30 | 12 | 18 |

Altogether, endocrine manipulation was applied to a total of 27 patients, but results are not yet available for 7 (Table 17). Seven, as noted above, with $R_f+$ tumors showed no evidence of disease progression in a 6- to 30-month period. One case with a $R_f-$ tumor, also, did not progress. There were five patients with advanced disease whose tumors were $R_f+$. Three had a total or partial regression of metastases, and in one the disease appeared

**Table 15**
**DISEASE-FREE**
**INTERVAL RELATED**
**TO STAGE OF DISEASE**
**AND $R_f$**

| Stage | $R_f$ | DFI in months (average) |
|-------|-------|-------------------------|
| 1 | + | 18.5 |
|   | − | 18 |
| 2 | + | 15.8 |
|   | − | 12.4 |
| 3a | + | 21 |
|    | − | 16 |
| 3b | + | — |
|    | − | 6 |
| 4 | + | 18 |
|   | − | 6 |
| X | + | 16.5 |
|   | − | — |

*Note:* Average R + = 17.5 months; R − = 12.4 months; DFI = disease free interval.

**Table 16**
**PATIENTS TREATED WITH ADJUVANT THERAPY**

| Type of therapy | $R_f$ | No. | No progression | Progression No. | % |
|-----------------|-------|-----|----------------|-----------------|---|
| Endocrine | + | 4 | 4 | 0 | 0 |
|           | − | 3 | 1 | 2 | 66 |
| Endocrine and X-ray | + | 2 | 2 | 0 | 0 |
|                     | − | 2 | 1 | 1 | 50 |
| Endocrine and chemotherapy | + | 1 | 1 | 0 | 0 |
|                            | − | 0 | 0 | 0 | 0 |
| Total |  | 12 | 9 | 3 |  |
| X-ray | + | 20 | 17 | 3 | 15 |
|       | − | 15 | 13 | 2 | 13 |
| X-ray and chemotherapy | + | 5 | 3 | 2 | 40 |
|                        | − | 7 | 4 | 3 | 42.8 |
| Chemotherapy | + | 23 | 21 | 2 | 8.6 |
|              | − | 40 | 36 | 4 | 10 |
| Total |  | 110 | 94 | 16 |  |

to be stabilized. Another patient progressed on endocrine treatment and then regressed with chemotherapy. On the other hand, only one of seven $R_f$− cases with advanced disease became stabilized, while six progressed with two dying. Although no conclusions of statistical significance can be made from this small series, nonetheless, it is quite evident that the $R_f$+ patients did far better than the $R_f$− cases.

**Table 17**
**ENDOCRINE MANIPULATION, ALONE OR ASSOCIATED, DURING THE COURSE OF THE DISEASE: RELATIONSHIP TO $R_f$**

| No. of cases | | No progression of disease | | Patients with advanced disease | | | |
|---|---|---|---|---|---|---|---|
| | | No. | Period (months) | No. | Total or partial regression | Stabilization | Progression of disease |
| $R_f$+ | 12 | 7 | 6—30 | 5 | 3 | 1 | 1 (regression with chemotherapy) |
| $R_f$− | 8 | 1 | 1 | 7 | 0 | 1 | 6 (2 ending with death) |
| Total | 20 | 8 | | 12 | 3 | 2 | 7 |

The advantages of planning endocrine therapy in patients with biochemically determined receptors, as compared to those of unknown receptor status, have been extensively reported.[19,51,52] Histochemical series, large enough to be of statistical significance, are now beginning to appear[15,36,53] and are further expanded elsewhere in these volumes. In our institution, comparison of results of histochemical and biochemical determinations has not been possible. However, others have published such data[14,27,54,55] and new, interesting data were presented at the Milan conference by Antoci et al.[13] and Wolf et al.[44]

It is worthwhile to emphasize the potential use of histochemistry on cytologic material[56] from both primary tumors as well as on secondary lesions from patients with advanced disease. To date it has been possible for us to evaluate the results of endocrine treatment in eight cases where $R_f$ was determined on this type of specimen. Of six $R_f$+ cases, five had a positive response. The other, after unsuccessful endocrine therapy, improved with chemotherapy. Two $R_f$− cases did not benefit from hormonal treatment.

Silfversward,[57] Tamura,[58] and Benyahia[59] applied the biochemical method to fine-needle aspirates, while Ide et al.[60] performed an interesting study on the in vivo response to tamoxifen on cytologic material obtained before and after a 7-day course of treatment, employing the Lee method. Mouriquand et al.[61] studied cells obtained by thin-needle aspiration prior to tamoxifen therapy and then on imprints from, subsequently, excised tumors. They noted a significant diminution of tamoxifen-induced fluorescence accompanied by ultrastructural evidence of nuclear damage in patients considered receptor-positive.

## V. CONCLUSIONS

The histochemical assay for the detection of putative estrogen receptors as described by Lee has now been tested by several investigators on tumors of the breast. In Italy, the data obtained by 13 independent laboratories were available for comparison at a meeting held in Milan in April 1983. When comparable, large, unselected series of cases were studied, the results appeared reproduceable and, for several parameters, not different from those obtained by biochemical receptor determinations. A large number of Italian pathologists are now engaged in verifying the clinical value of the method under the auspices of the Italian Society of Hospital Pathologists. As pointed out by Pertschuk et al. in this work, the binding sites revealed by histochemistry may be different than those demonstrated biochemically. However, clinical response to endocrine therapy may be similarly predicted.

The histochemical method may readily be performed in most laboratories of anatomic pathology and mastered by personnel adequately experienced in breast cancer morphology as well as fluorescence microscopy. There is abundant evidence that the size of breast cancers at the time of first diagnosis is decreasing. Thus, the number of cases with a quantity of tumor tissue adequate for biochemical assay can be expected to decrease. In addition, in Italy as well as in many other countries, only a few institutions have the required facilities for performance of the biochemical assay. Improper selection of material for biochemical assay, failure of refrigeration, and delay in transportation of specimens requiring shipment to a reference center may be responsible at times for erroneous biochemical results. Results of histochemistry can be available on the same day as surgery is performed and can also be applied to the study of cytologic material obtained from patients with metastatic lesions.

In our series, the rate of positivity was 57.5% of 356 primary tumors. The highest positivity was found between 45 and 49 years of age and after age 55. Not previously emphasized and, therefore, somewhat surprising was an abrupt decrease in the number of positive cases between ages 50 and 54. This inverted distribution during this period of life requires further investigation.

Some other interesting facts have emerged from this study. The percentage of positive tumors of small size was higher than that of the overall series (65.4%). The strange relationship between $R_f$ and tumor size during the perimenopausal period observed by us also requires further evaluation. It is of interest that our stage 1 patients were more often positive, suggesting a more favorable prognosis. The high proportion of positive cases where the tumor margin was irregular may be related to the extensive criteria we use in evaluating this parameter. The distribution of $R_f$ in the various tumor types does not differ from other reports. The almost constant positivity of lobular carcinomas at all ages and the high rate of positive ductal carcinomas in the older age groups are worth noting.

Clinical follow-up has been obtained on slightly over 50% of our cases but is only in a preliminary phase at this writing. Progression of disease was less common in $R_f+$ women. Nine deaths have occurred in this brief time period and only three in the $R_f+$ group. The longer disease-free interval and the lower rate of recurrence and/or metastases suggests a better prognosis in $R_f+$ cases and is further suggested by $R_f$ distribution by tumor size and disease stage. The lack of disease progression in the few positive cases treated with adjunct endocrine therapy, compared with the percentage of positive and negative cases progressing on nonhormonal therapy, together with the regression or stabilization apparent in $R_f+$ cases with advanced disease, are all highly suggestive of a positive correlation between histochemically determined positivity and response to endocrine therapy. Since more than one half of breast cancers are $R_f+$, a better prognosis might be obtained by the more frequent employment of adjunct endocrine therapy. Finally, the application of the method to cytologic material appears to represent a valuable tool both as a complement to the assay of tissue sections and as the only potential, available method in many patients with advanced disease.

## ACKNOWLEDGMENTS

The authors are grateful for the cooperation of Drs. M. A. De Bernardi and G. Vitullo. They also thank Mr. C. Forese and all colleagues at the Busto Arsizio Hospital. Special thanks are due to Dr. E. Bossi of the Centro di Calcolo dell 'Università Cattolica, Busto Arsizio.

# REFERENCES

1. **Facente, L. F., Carnaghi, P. L., and Lampertico, P.,** Epidemiologia dei tumori della mammella in una città di 80000 abitanti nee corso degli ultimi trenta anni, *Pathologica,* 74, 593, 1982.
2. **Cislaghi, C., De Carli, A., Morosini, P., and Puntoni, R.,** Atlante della mortalità per tumori in Italia triennio 1970—72, in *Lega Italiana per la Lotta Contro i Tumori,* Roma, 1978.
3. **Berrino, F., Crosignani, P., Riboli, E., and Viganò, C.,** Epidemiologia dei tumori maligni: incidenza e mortalità in Provincia di Varese 1976—1977, in *Notizie Sanità; Mensile e Cura dell' Assessorato Regionale alla Sanità della Regione Lombardia,* Scotti Editore, Milano, Luglio, 1981.
4. **Foncam, I.,** Tumori della mammella: protocollo di trattamento, Milano, Giugno, 1979.
5. **Pertschuk, L. P., Tobin, E. N., Brigati, D. J., Kim, D. S., Bloom, N. D., Gaetjens, E., Berman, P. J., Carter, A. C., and Degenshein, G. A.,** Immunofluorescent detection of estrogen receptors in breast cancer, *Cancer,* 41, 907, 1978.
6. **Nenci, I.,** Citochimica dei Recettori Ormonali nei tumori ormono responsivi. Il ruolo del patologo, *Pathologica,* 71, 431, 1979.
7. **Lee, S. H.,** Cancer cell estrogen receptor of human mammary carcinoma, *Cancer,* 44, 1, 1979.
8. **Lampertico, P.,** Determinazione dei Recettori Ormonali in 13 laboratori, *Istocitopatologia,* 6, 47, 1984.
9. **Gambacorta, M.,** Interpretazione dei risultati e formulazione della risposta, *Istocitopatologia,* 6, 33, 1984.
10. **Lunetta, Q.,** Presupposti per una corretta interpretazione dei risultati, *Istocitopatologia,* 6, 41, 1984.
11. **Stagni, F., De Bernardi, M. A., and Lampertico, P.,** Metodica di base, *Istocitopatologia,* 6, 11, 1984.
12. **Pertschuk, L. P., Tobin, E. H., Gaetjens, E., Carter, A. C., Degenshein, G. A., Bloom, N. D., and Brigati, D. J.,** Histochemical assay of estrogen and progesterone receptors in breast cancer: correlation with biochemical assay and patients response to endocrine therapies, *Cancer,* 46, 2896, 1980.
13. **Antoci, B., Costantini, M., Rocco, M., and Pizzolitto, S.,** Studio dei recettori steroidei nel carcinoma della mammella: I° esperienza dell 'Istituto di Anatomia Patologica dell 'Ospedale Civile di Udine su 180 casi; II° comparazione tra "Metodo radiometrico e quello di istofluorescenza", *Istocitopatologia,* 6, 17, 1984.
14. **Meijer, C. J. L. M., Van Marle, Y., Persign, Y. P., Van Niewenhuizen, W., Baak, Y. P. A., Boon, M. E., and Lindeman, Y.,** Estrogen receptors in human breast cancer. II. Correlation between the histochemical method and biochemical assay, *Virchows Arch.,* 40, 27, 1982.
15. **Pertschuk, L. P.,** Comparison of morphologic and biochemical steroid binding assay in breast cancer; clinical correlation, method of quantification, *Istocitopatologia,* 6, 67, 1984.
16. **Gambacorta, M.,** Rapporto tra neoplasia e stroma nei tumori mammari, presented at the Milan Conf., April 16, 1983.
17. **Lesser, M. L., Rosen, P. P., Senie, R. T., Duthie, K., Menendez-Botet, C., and Schwartz, M. K.,** Estrogen and progesterone receptors in breast carcinoma: correlations with epidemiology and pathology, *Cancer,* 48, 299, 1981.
18. **Elwood, Y. N. and Godolphin, W.,** Oestrogen receptors in breast tumors: associations with age, menopausal status and epidemiological and clinical features in 735 patients, *Br. J. Cancer,* 42, 635, 1980.
19. **McGuire, W. L. and Horwitz, B.,** Progesterone receptors in breast cancer, in *Hormones, Receptors and Breast Cancer,* McGuire, W. L., Ed., Raven Press, New York, 1978.
20. **Chabon, A. B., Goldberg, Y. D., and Venet, L.,** Carcinoma of the breast: interrelationships among histopathologic features, estrogen receptors activity and age of the patient, *Hum. Pathol.,* 14, 368, 1983.
21. **Sugano, H., Sakamoto, G., Sakamoto, A., Nomura, Y., Takatani, O., and Matsumoto, K.,** Hormone receptors and histopathology in Japanese breast cancer, in *Hormones, Receptors and Breast Cancer,* McGuire, W. L., Ed., Raven Press, New York, 1978.
22. **Fisher, E. R., Redmond, C. K., Liu, H., Rockette, H., Fischer, B., and Coll. NSABP Investigators,** Correlation of estrogen receptor and pathologic characteristics of invasive breast cancer, *Cancer,* 45, 349, 1980.
23. **Parl, F. F. and Wagner, R. K.,** The histopathological evaluation of human breast cancer in correlation with estrogen receptors values, *Cancer,* 46, 362, 1980.
24. **Pertschuk, L. P., Tobin, E. H., Tanapat, P. et al.,** Histochemical analysis of steroid hormone receptors in breast and prostatic carcinoma, *J. Histochem. Cytochem.,* 28, 799, 1980.
25. **Jacobs, S. R., Wolfson, W. L., Cheng, L., and Lewin, K. Y.,** Cytochemical and competitive protein binding assays for estrogen receptor in breast disease, *Cancer,* 51, 1671, 1983.
26. **Paulsen, S. M., Johansen, P., Rasmussen, K. S., and Mygind, H.,** Histokemisk påvisning af Østrogemreceptore ved mammakarcinom, *Usegkr. Laeg.,* 143, 3119, 1981.
27. **O'Connell, M. D. and Said, Y. W.,** Estrogen receptors in carcinoma of the breast. A comparison of the dextran-coated charcoal, immunofluorescent, and immunoperoxidase technics, *Am. J. Clin. Pathol.,* 80, 1, 1983.

28. **Shimizu, M., Wayima, O., Miura, M., and Katayama, I.,** Pap immunoperoxidase method demonstrating endogenous estrogen in breast carcinomas, *Cancer,* 52, 486, 1983.

29. **Taylor, C. R., Cooper, C. L., Kurman, R. Y., Goebelsmann, U., and Markland, F. S.,** Detection of estrogen receptor in breast and endometrial carcinoma by the immunoperoxidase technique, *Cancer,* 47, 2634, 1981.

30. **Nenci, I., Piffanelli, A., Beccati, M. D., and Lanza, G.,** *In vivo* and *in vitro* immunofluorescent approach to the physiopathology of estradiol kinetics in target cells, *J. Steroid Biochem.,* 7, 883, 1976.

31. **Nenci, I., Beccati, M. D., and Arslan-Pagnini, C.,** Estrogen receptors and post-receptor markers in human breast cancer: a reappraisal, *Tumori,* 64, 161, 1978.

32. **Nenci, I., Marchetti, E., Marzola, A., Fabris, G., and Rotola, A.,** Bases et applications de la cytochimie des récepteurs stéroidiens, *Int. J. Breast Mammary Pathol. Senol.,* 1, 15, 1982.

33. **Lee, S. H.,** Sex steroid hormone receptors in mammary carcinoma, in *Diagnostic Immunohistochemistry,* De Lellis, R. A., Ed., Masson, Paris, 1981.

34. **Lee, S. H.,** Uterine epithelial and eosinophil estrogen receptors in rats during the estrous cycle, *Histochemistry,* 74, 443, 1982.

35. **Berger, G., Frappart, L., Depardon, Y., and Bremond, A.,** Etude histochimique des récepteurs d'estradiol et de la progestérone à l'aide des complexes de Lee dans 40 cancers mammaires. Correlations avec la différenciation et le type histopathologique, *Int. J. Breast Mammary Pathol. Senol.,* 1, 19, 1982.

36. **Pertschuk, L. P., Eisenberg, K. B., Leo, V. C., Carter, A. C., and Gaetjens, E.,** Correlation of estrogen binding by histochemistry in breast cancer with clinical response to hormonal therapies, *Lab. Invest.,* 46, 165A, 1982.

37. **Zaroli, S., Signorelli, E., Stagni, F., and Lampertico, P.,** The renal adenocarcinoma: epidemiological, clinical, pathological and cultural considerations based on 117 cases, *Pathologica,* 76, 169, 1984.

38. **Roberts, A. N. and Hannel, R.,** Oestrogen receptor assay and morphology of breast cancer, *Pathology,* 13, 317, 1981.

39. **Rosen, P. P., Menendez-Botet, C. J., Senie, R. T., Schwartz, M. K., Schottenfeld, D., and Farr, G. H.,** Estrogen receptor protein (ERP) and the histopathology of human mammary carcinoma, in *Hormones, Receptors, and Breast Cancer,* McGuire, W. L., Ed., Raven Press, New York, 1978.

40. **UICC,** *TNM Classification of Malignant Tumors,* 3rd ed., Geneva, 1978.

41. **Fisher, E. R., Gregorio, R. M., Fisher, B., with the assistance of Redmond, C., Vellios, F., Sommer, S. C., and Cooperating Investigators,** The pathology of invasive breast cancer. A syllabus derived from findings of the national surgical adjuvant breast project (Prot. n. 4), *Cancer,* 36, 1, 1975.

42. **Hull, D. F., Clark, G. M., Osborne, C. K., Chamness, G. C., Knight, W. A., and McGuire, W. L.,** Multiple estrogen receptor assays in human breast cancer, *Cancer Res.,* 43, 413, 1983.

43. **Underwood, J. C. E.,** Oestrogen receptors in human breast cancer: review of histopathological correlations and critique of histochemical methods, *Diagn. Histopathol.,* 6, 1, 1983.

44. **Wolf, D., Gion, M., Melia, M., and Forti, E.,** Determinazione citochimica dei recettori per estrogeni e progesterone nelle neoplasie mammarie; correlazioni cliniche e primo confronto con un metodo radiometrico, *Istocitopatologia,* 6, 55, 1984.

45. **Schenck, U., Burger, G., Eiermann, W., and Peters-Welte, C.,** Correlation between cytomorphological and hormone-receptor evaluation of breast carcinoma, *Abstracts, 12th European Congr. of Cytology,* Paris, 1983.

46. **Reguzzoni, G., Stagni, F., and Lampertico, P.,** Risultati preliminari della correlazione clinica tra assetto recettoriale e follow up, *Istocitopatologia,* 6, 73, 1984.

47. **Harland, R. N. L., Barnes, D. M., Howell, A., Ribeiro, G. G., Taylor, J., and Sellwood, R. A.,** Variation of receptor status in cancer of the breast, *Br. J. Cancer,* 47, 511, 1983.

48. **Crowe, J. P., Hubay, C. A., Pearson, O. N. et al.,** Estrogen receptor status as a prognostic indicator for stage 1 breast cancer patients, *Breast Cancer Res. Treat.,* 2, 171, 1982.

49. **Heise, E. and Gorlish, M.,** Estradiol receptor activity in human breast cancer, disease free interval and survival time, *Ant. Cancer Res.,* 2, 33, 1982.

50. **Kinne, D. W., Ashikari, R., Butler, A., Menendez-Botet, C., Rosen, P. P., and Schwartz, M.,** Estrogen receptor protein in breast cancer as a predictor of recurrence, *Cancer,* 47, 2364, 1981.

51. **Nomura, Y., Yamagata, J., Kondo, H., Kanda, K., and Takenaka, K.,** Clinical usefulness of estrogen receptor assay in early and advanced breast cancer, in *Hormones, Receptors, and Breast Cancer,* McGuire, W. L., Ed., Raven Press, New York, 1978.

52. **Matsumoto, K., Ochi, H., Nomura, Y., Takatami, O., Izuo, M., Okamoto, R., and Sugano, H.,** Progesterone and estrogen receptors in Japanese breast cancer, in *Hormones, Receptors, and Breast Cancer,* McGuire, W. L., Ed., Raven Press, New York, 1978.

53. **Yao, X., Lee, S. H., and Tourville, D. R.,** A histochemical technique for the demonstration of estrogen receptor in human breast cancer, *Istocitopatologia,* 6, 5, 1984.

54. **Tominaga, T., Kimatura, M., Saito, T., Itoh, I., and Takikawa, H.,** Comparative histochemical and biochemical assays of estrogen receptors in breast cancer patients, *Gann,* 72, 6, 1981.

55. **Eusebi, V., Cerasoli, P. T., Guidelli-Guidi, S., Grilli, S., Bussolati, G., and Azzopardi, J. G.,** A two-stage immunocytochemical method for oestrogen receptor analysis: correlation with morphological parameters of breast carcinoma, *Tumori,* 67, 315, 1981.

56. **Curtin, C. T., Pertschuk, L. P., and Mitchell, V.,** Histochemical determination of estrogen and progesterone binding in fine needle aspirates of breast cancer: correlation with conventional biochemical assays, *Acta Cytol.,* 26(6), 841, 1982.

57. **Silfversward, C. and Humla, S.,** Estrogen receptor analysis on needle aspirates from human mammary carcinoma, *Acta Cytol.,* 24(1), 54, 1980.

58. **Tamura, H., Raam, S., Nemeth, E., and Cohen, J.,** Immunohistochemical detection of estrogen receptors in human breast carcinoma using antireceptor antibodies: its application to cytologic material, *Lab. Invest.,* 46, 82A, 1982.

59. **Benyahia, B., Magdelenat, H., Zajdela, A., and Vilcoq, J. B.,** Ponction-aspiration à l'aiguille fine et dosage des récepteurs d'oestrogénes dans le cancer du sein, *Bull. Cancer (Paris),* 69, 5, 456, 1982.

60. **Ide, P., Billiet, G., and Bonte, J.,** Etude de l'aspect cytologique et des modifications de l'intensité de la fluorescence de cellules tumorales mammaires humaines après sept jours de traitement au tamoxiféne, *Int. J. Breast Mammary Pathol. Senol.,* 1, 33, 1982.

61. **Mouriquand, J., Mouriquand, C., Sage, J. C., Jacrot, M., Sael, S., and Gabelle, P.,** Etude cytologique de la fluorescence du tamoxiféne chez des femmes porteuses de cancer du sein, traitées: un marqueur de l'hormonodépendance, *Int. J. Breast Mammary Pathol. Senol.,* 1, 29, 1983.

Chapter 6

# HOW TO VALIDATE HISTOCHEMICAL TECHNIQUES AS PREDICTORS OF HORMONAL RESPONSE

**Wedad Hanna and Kathleen I. Pritchard**

## TABLE OF CONTENTS

I.      Introduction ................................................................. 86

II.     Materials and Method ....................................................... 86
        A.      Histochemical Technique .......................................... 86

III.    Controls .................................................................... 86

IV.     Statistical Analysis ........................................................ 87
        A.      Correlation of the Histochemical and Biochemical Assay ............... 87
        B.      Response Criteria ................................................ 87
        C.      Results .......................................................... 87
                1.      Distribution of the Histochemical Assay ................... 87
                2.      Correlation of Histochemical and Biochemical Assay ........... 87
                3.      Correlation of Results of the Histochemical Assay with Patient's
                        Response to Endocrine Therapy ............................... 88

V.      Discussion ................................................................. 88

References .................................................................... 90

# I. INTRODUCTION

There is controversy as to the validity of histochemical techniques to localize estrogen receptors (ER) in human breast cancer. Using an estrogen BSA FITC complex, several groups[1-3] have attempted to evaluate the presence of steroid receptors at the cellular level in frozen sections or in cell suspensions of human breast cancer.[4] Originally, Pertschuk et al. and Lee et al. suggested that their fluoresceinated compounds localized estrogen receptor. Other groups have shown by extensive biochemical tests, however, that the positive fluorescence seen using fluoresceinated estradiol in a histochemical technique is not due to interaction with type 1 estrogen receptors.[5,6] Using a fluoresceinated estradiol, we find that we are seeing differential staining and that there is a mixture of positive and negative cells in each of a large number of tumor specimens.[7] Therefore, we feel, as do other groups working in this area, that the histochemical reaction is specific.[8,9] Whether these fluoresceinated tracers are localizing types 1 or so-called type 2 receptors[10] or other classes of estrogen binding proteins is not clear. It is our feeling, however, that the "gold standard" for histochemical techniques to localize estrogen receptors should be their ability to predict clinical response to hormone manipulation rather than simply their correlation with standard biochemical techniques for measuring receptors. Therefore, we have tried not only to correlate the results of our fluoresceinated technique with standard biochemical assays, but, also, to get as much information as possible about the ability of both types of receptor assays to predict for hormone response in the clinical setting.

# II. MATERIALS AND METHOD

Between November 1, 1979 and January 1, 1983, we examined 286 consecutive specimens of human breast cancer from Women's College Hospital, Toronto, Canada. At the time of the quick section, six addition sections, 6 to 8 μm thick, were cut and stored at $-70°C$ for no more than a month. Adjacent areas from the breast tumor are also immediately frozen and sent to Dr. Elizabeth Mobbs, for the biochemical evaluation of the receptors, using the dextran-coated charcoal method.

## A. Histochemical Technique

1. One slide was stained with hematoxylin and eosin.
2. Two others were rehydrated by brief immersion in phosphate-buffered saline pH 7.4 (PBS) and then dried.
3. The slides were incubated with the tracer, fluoresceinated estradiol*, for 1 hr in a humid chamber at 4°C.
4. The slides were then washed three times at 5-min intervals in PBS.
5. They were then dried and mounted with glycerol.

# III. CONTROLS

For every new batch of the tracer, we used the following controls:

1. Positive controls: cryostat sections of human endometrium and myometrium; and cryostat sections of uterus from oophorectomized Sprague-Dawley rats.

---

* This hydrophyllic fluorescent estrogen reagent, 17β-estradiol-6-CMO BSA-FITC, was the tracer used. It was first purchased directly from Dr. Lee at St. Raphael's Hospital, and as of January 1, 1981 it was bought from Zeus Scientific, Inc., (Fluoro-Cep™).

2.   Negative controls: cryostat sections of human skeletal muscle, lung, and/or lymph nodes.

Blocking with unlabeled estradiol was also carried out. DES was diluted to $2 \times 10^{-4}\,M$ in PBS containing 0.5 m$M$ dithiothreitol and 10% glycerin. The slides were then examined using a fluorescent microscope and the following points were evaluated:

1.   The corresponding H and E section was used to evaluate the tumor type and to estimate the percentage of tumor vs. stroma.
2.   According to the percentage of cells with positive fluorescence, the tumors were divided into three groups: (1) definitely positive for estrogen binding sites — 90% or more positive; (2) definitely negative for estrogen binding sites — 10% or less positive; and (3) intermediate groups — 10 to 90% positive.
3.   The intensity of the fluorescence was recorded as to + to + + +, using the fluorescence observed in adjacent normal ducts as the + + level.
4.   The intensity of the fluorescence was recorded as to + to + + +, using the fluorescence observed in adjacent normal ducts as the + + level.

## IV. STATISTICAL ANALYSIS

### A. Correlation of the Histochemical and Biochemical Assay

With the experience gained from correlating our first 59 fluoresceinated assays with standard biochemical assay,[7] we chose to correlate the values of the biochemical assay with the results of the histochemical technique for tumors in group 1 and 2 (those with 90% or more positive cells and those with 10% or less positive cells) using a chi-squared table, the reason being the absence of an acceptable cutoff point for negative and positive in the intermediate group.

### B. Response Criteria

The response criteria used to define "objective regression" of tumor were those of Hayward et al.[11]

### C. Results

*1. Distribution of the Histochemical Assay*

The 286 patients were divided according to the results of the histochemical techniques, into three groups, which are shown:

| | | |
|---|---|---|
| Positive — 90% of cells are positive | 77 | patients |
| Negative — 10% of cells are positive | 120 | patients |
| Intermediate group | 87 | patients |

*2. Correlation of Histochemical and Biochemical Assay*

The results of comparing histochemical and biochemical assays in group 1 and 2 indicate that a tumor which will be labeled as positive or negative for estrogen binding by the histochemical technique will be similarly called by the biochemical assay, $p < 0.001$, as shown in Table 1. Note from Table 1 that using the histochemical technique, there were 120/286 patients which are negative for the receptor, i.e., 41%. Out of those 43/120 were ER positive by the biochemical assay (65% concordance). On the other hand, out of 79 ER positive by the histochemical assay, only 21 were labeled ER negative by the receptor biochemical assay (75% concordance).

**Table 1**
**BIOCHEMICAL ASSAY**

(Standard)

| Histochemical technique | ER + | ER − | Total |
|---|---|---|---|
| ER + | 59 (a) | 20 (c) | 79 |
| Er − | 43 (b) | 77 (d) | 120 |
| $p < 0.001$ | 102 | 97 | 199 |

Since there is no acceptable cutoff point for the positive and negative cases in the intermediate group, correlation of the results of these two techniques was not attempted for this group.

*3. Correlation of Results of the Histochemical Assay with Patient's Response to Endocrine Therapy*

Of the 286 patients in our study for whom the receptors were histochemically evaluated, the vast majority were unevaluable for response to hormonal therapy. The records for 37 patients were not available for follow-up. Of the remaining 249, 182 have not yet developed recurrent disease. Of the 67 patients who have developed recurrent disease, 29 had their recurrence either surgically excised (26) or radiated (3). Six were lost to follow-up after recurrence and four received no systemic therapy of any type. Of the remaining 28 patients, 9 were treated with chemotherapy alone, while 4 were treated with chemotherapy plus hormonal therapy, thus, making them unassessable for response to hormonal therapy. Of the 15 patients on hormonal therapy, 4 are too early to assess. The response of the remaining 11 patients, who were all treated with tamoxifen, showed 6 failures and 5 objective responses. The results of their receptor assays by the biochemical and histochemical techniques are shown in Tables 2 and 3.

Although there is no known cutoff point for the intermediate group, one would expect a tumor with 50% positive cells and + + intensity of the fluorescence to respond to hormonal manipulation. As shown in Tables 2 and 3, the response was predicted correctly in 8/11 cases by the histochemical technique (cases 2, 3, 4, 5, 7, 8, 9, and 11), compared to 6/11 by the biochemical technique.

## V. DISCUSSION

The evaluation of steroid receptors in human breast cancer has become important in the management of breast cancer patients, both in guiding treatment decisions and as a prognostic factor.[12] The difficulties encountered with expensive and meticulous techniques such as the biochemical assay have stimulated several groups[13-16] to supplement this method by histochemical techniques which attempt to localize estrogen receptors at the cellular level. In this report, we have not addressed what these histochemical tracers are localizing, but we have examined the correlation between histochemical and biochemical techniques, and, most important, the ability of the histochemical technique to predict response to therapy. Tumor heterogeneity for biological markers is a well-known phenomenon in cancer.[18] It becomes apparent, using histochemical techniques, that in any breast cancer there are mixtures of positive and negative cells. The combination of histochemical and biochemical receptor techniques may help to overcome the problems posed by this tumor heterogeneity.

## Table 2
## FAILURES (PROGRESSIVE DISEASE)

### ER Status

| Patients | Biochemical assay (fmol/mg protein) | Histochemical assay % of positive cells and intensity of fluorescence |
|---|---|---|
| Cases | | |
| (1) Mrs. G[a] | 1° 121 | 1° Not available |
| | 2° 4, 27, 11, 15, | 2° (No. 6) 25% + + |
| | 52, 38, 100 | (No. 2) 50% + + |
| (2) Mrs. H | 1° 69 | 1° 10% + + |
| (3) Mrs. R | 1° 12 | 1° 10% + |
| (4) Mrs. St | 1° 127 | 1° 0% |
| (5) Mrs. S | 1° 10 | 1° 10% + + |
| | 2° 24 | |
| (6) Mrs. B | 1° 27 | 1° 50% + + |

[a]   2° are multiple skin nodules which were excised at different dates.

## Table 3
## OBJECTIVE RESPONSE TO TAMOXIFEN

### ER Status

| Patients | Biochemical assay (fmol/mg protein) | Histochemical assay % of positive cells and intensity of fluorescence |
|---|---|---|
| Cases | | |
| (7) Mrs. L | 1° 142 | 50% + + |
| (8) Mrs. M | 1° 25 | 50% + + |
| (9) Mrs. D | 1° 125 | 100% + + |
| (10) Mrs. Sm | 1° 39 | 2° (1st nodule) 10% + + |
| | 2° 49, 193 | |
| (11) Mrs. Ge[a] | 1° 323 | 50% + + |
| | | 40% + |
| | | 10% − ve |

[a]   Illustrates the marked heterogeneity of a tumor.

Problems in evaluating the results of the histochemical technique come from the fact that there is no established cutoff point to distinguish between negative and positive tumors using the percentage of positive cells and the intensity of fluorescence. This also hampers the correlation between the histochemical and biochemical techniques. This problem has not been well addressed in any previous studies. Perstchuk et al. took 20% positive cells as the cutoff point for positivity, while Lee et al. used 50% as the positive value. These values are used without incorporation of the intensity of the fluorescence. Meijer et al.[19] on the other hand, considered a tumor negative when:

1.     The presence of 1+ intensity, irrespective of the percentage of cells
2.     10% or less tumor cells are negative

We believe that, as with the biochemical assay, the patient's response to therapy should be the major guideline in deciding a cutoff point for positive and negative cases using the histochemical techniques. However, from our experience as from Meijer's work, we found that by the histochemical technique, tumors with less than 10% positive cells tend to correlate with estrogen receptor negativity by biochemical techniques, while tumors with 50% or more positive cells correlated with biochemical estrogen receptor positivity. The intensity of the fluorescence is also of significance regardless of the percentage of positive cells; 1 + intensity is always associated with negative biochemical receptor status. Looking at Tables 2 and 3, it is interesting to note that the tumor with 50% + + cells may have different biochemical ER contents, as shown in cases 1, 6, 7, and 8, and also different responses to hormonal therapy. These results stress the need for the combination of chemotherapy and hormonal therapy in such cases. Case 11 illustrates the marked heterogeneity of a tumor and the variation in the intensity of fluorescence which may reflect different receptor contents. Also, it shows the difficulties in interpretation encountered in the histochemical technique with 50% of cells showing + + intensity, 40% showing one + intensity, and 10% negative cells. Statistical analysis using the chi-square test showed a $p$ value of $\leq 0.001$ when correlating the histochemical and biochemical techniques. This correlation suggests that using fluoresceinated estrogen at the cellular level, one is either localizing the true estrogen receptor or an estrogen binding site that is closely associated with the receptor. The binding sites seen with the histochemical technique are probably not the type 1 receptor, but may represent a site that correlated closely with it.

The number of cases that we have available for correlation with the clinical response is very small, however, the histochemical technique has predicted the response to endocrine therapy correctly in 8 out of 11 patients, compared to 6 out of 11 patients predicted correctly by the biochemical assay. We strongly feel that correlation of the results of the histochemical technique with the patient's response to hormonal therapy is very important, in order to establish the value of the histochemical technique and help to define criteria of positivity. Critical evaluation of response to endocrine therapy in a much larger number of patients and continued correlation with histochemical and biochemical techniques are required. Over the next few years, many of the patients we have assayed, at the time of primary surgery, will develop recurrences and should provide further data of this type.

# REFERENCES

1. **Lee, S. H.,** Cellular estrogen and progesterone receptors in mammary carcinoma, *Am. J. Clin. Pathol.,* 73(3), 323, 1980.
2. **Pertschuk, L. P., Gaetjens, E., Carter, A. C., Brigati, D. J., Kim, D. S., and Tobin, E. H.,** Histochemistry of steroid receptors in breast cancer: an overview, *Ann. Clin. Lab. Sci.,* 9(3), 219, 1979.
3. **Walker, R. A., Cove, D. H., and Howell, A.,** Histochemical detection of oestrogen receptor in human breast carcinomas, *Lancet,* 1, 171, 1980.
4. **Nenci, I., Beccati, M. D., Piffanelli, A., and Lanza, G.,** Detection and dynamic localization of estradiol-receptor complexes in intact target cells by immunofluorescence technique, *J. Steroid Biochem.,* 7, 505, 1976.
5. **Chamness, G. C., Mercer, W. D., and McGuire, W. L.,** Are histochemical methods for estrogen receptor valid, *J. Histochem. Cytochem.,* 28, 792, 1980.
6. **DeSombre, E. R., Carbone, P. P., Jensen, E. V., McGuire, W. L., Wells, S. A., Jr., Wittliff, J. L., and Lipsett, M. B.,** Steroid receptors in breast cancer (report of a consensus-development meeting, NIH, June, 1979), *N. Engl. J. Med.,* 301, 1011, 1979.
7. **Hanna, W., Ryder, D. E., and Mobbs, B. G.,** Cellular localization of estrogen binding sites in human breast cancer, *Am. J. Clin. Pathol.,* 77(4), 391, 1982.

8. **van Marle, J., Lindeman, J., Ariëns, A. Th., Labruyère, W., and van Weeren-Kramer, J.,** Estrogen receptors in human breast cancer. I. Specificity of the histochemical localization of estrogen receptor using an estrogen-albumin FITC complex, *Virchows Arch. (Cell Pathol.),* 40, 17, 1982.

9. **Lee, S. H.,** The histochemistry of estrogen receptors, *Histochemistry,* 71, 491, 1981.

10. **Clark, J. H., Hardin, J. W., Upchurch, S., and Eriksson, H.,** Heterogeneity of estrogen binding sites in the cytosol of the rat uterus, *J. Biol. Chem.,* 253, 7630, 1978.

11. **Hayward, J. L., Meakin, J. W., and Stewart, H. J.,** Assessment of response and recurrence in breast cancer, *Semin. Oncol.,* 5, 445, 1978.

12. **McGuire, W. L., Horwitz, K. B., Zava, D. T., Garola, R. E., and Chamness, G. C.,** Hormones in breast cancer: update 1978, *Metabolism,* 28, 487, 1978.

13. **Barrows, G. H., Stroupe, S. B., and Riehm, J. D.,** Nuclear uptake of a 17β estradiol-fluorescence derivative as a marker of estrogen dependance, *Am. J. Clin. Pathol.,* 73, 330, 1980.

14. **Dandliker, W. B., Brawn, R. J., Hso, M.-L., Brawn, P. N., Levin, J., Meyers, C. Y., and Kolb, V. M.,** Investigation of hormone-receptor interactions by means of fluorescence labeling, *Cancer Res.,* 38, 4212, 1978.

15. **Lee, S. H.,** Cancer cell estrogen receptor of human mammary carcinoma, *Cancer,* 44, 1, 1979.

16. **Mercer, W. D., Lippman, M. E., Wahl, T. M., Carlson, C. A., Wahl, D. A., Lezotte, D., and Teague, P. O.,** The use of immunocytochemical techniques for the detection of steroid hormones in breast cancer cells, *Cancer,* 46, 2859, 1980.

17. **Fisher, B., Gunduz, N., Zheng, S., and Saffer, E. A.,** Fluoresceinated estrone binding by human and mouse breast cancer cells, *Cancer Res.,* 42, 540, 1982.

18. **Marx, J. L.,** Tumours: a mixed bag of cells, *Science,* 215, 275, 1982.

19. **Meijer, C. J. L. M., van Marle, J., Persijn, J. P., van Niewenhuizen, W., Baak, J. P. A., Boon, M. E., and Lindeman, J.,** Estrogen receptors in human breast cancer. II. Correlations between the histochemical method and biochemical assay, *Virchows Arch. (Cell Pathol.),* 40, 27, 1982.

Chapter 7

# LOCALIZATION OF STEROID BINDING IN PROSTATIC CARCINOMA BY HISTOCHEMISTRY: THERAPEUTIC IMPLICATIONS*

**Louis P. Pertschuk, Richard J. Macchia, and Karen B. Eisenberg**

## TABLE OF CONTENTS

I.       Introduction ............................................................... 94

II.      Methodology for Histochemical Androgen Binding Assay ...................... 94

III.     Specificity Studies with Fluorescent Androgens ............................... 95

IV.     Comparison of Histochemical and Biochemical Androgen Binding Assays ...... 95

V.      Cytoplasmic vs. Nuclear Androgen Binding .................................. 95

VI.     Correlation of Histochemical Androgen Binding Assay with Clinical Response to Endocrine Therapy ....................................................... 98

VII.     Estrogen Binding in Prostatic Carcinoma .................................... 103

VIII.    Other Histochemical Studies of Steroid Binding in the Prostate ................ 104

IX.     Studies of Prostatic Carcinoma with Monoclonal Antibodies to Estrogen Receptor ................................................................ 104

X.      Multiplicity of Estrogen Binding Sites in Prostatic Carcinoma ................ 104

XI.     Advantages of Histochemical Steroid Binding Assays in Prostatic Carcinoma .. 105

XII.     Androgen Binding in Prostatic Disease Other than Carcinoma ................ 106

XIII.    Detection of Endogenous Steroid Bound In Vivo ............................. 107

XIV.    Relationship between Prostatic Acid Phosphatase and Androgen Binding by Histochemistry ......................................................... 107

XV.     The Nature of the Binding Revealed by Histochemical Steroid Binding Assays in Prostate ............................................................... 108

Acknowledgments ............................................................... 108

References ...................................................................... 109

\*   Supported by USPHS Grant No. CA25760 from the National Prostatic Cancer Project, NCI.

# I. INTRODUCTION

Huggins and Hodges[1] were the first to report that a sizeable proportion of men with advanced prostatic carcinoma responded satisfactorily to endocrine manipulation. Their findings were corroborated in several large-scale clinical trials.[2,3] Since then, additive and/or ablative hormonal therapies have been prime weapons in the treatment of metastatic prostatic malignancy.

In 1971, Hansson and colleagues[4] detected high-affinity, low-capacity, tissue-specific androgen receptors (AR) in specimens of prostatic tissue and their results have been duplicated and their technique refined by numerous workers.[5-23] More recently, with the synthesis of androgenic ligands with limited ability to bind to testosterone binding globulin (TeBG),[11,24] there is increasing evidence that men with AR-positive tumors are more likely to respond to hormonal treatment than are men with AR-negative neoplasms.[23,34]

In spite of this knowledge, biochemical AR determinations have never achieved wide popularity as an aid in the planning of rational therapy for cases of advanced prostate cancer, and such patients are usually selected for hormone therapy solely on an empirical basis. Indeed, the study of AR in prostate cancer is in its infancy when compared to estrogen receptors (ER) in breast cancer. Mainwaring has summarized some of the reasons for this state of affairs.[35] Prostatic carcinoma specimens not infrequently are composed of a heterogeneous conglomerate of benign as well as malignant cellular components. Since homogenization is a prerequisite to biochemical AR assay, there is no way to ascertain whether any receptor that may be measurable is derived from the benign or the malignant tissue elements. Another problem is that it is difficult to homogenize tissue with a fibromuscular stroma in that this step may result in the production of heat. This can be minimized by frequent cooling of the specimen during the homogenization process. Because many prostate tissue samples are secured by electrocautery, there may be damage to heat-labile AR. Furthermore, the diagnosis of prostatic cancer is frequently made by needle biopsy, consequently, the amount of tissue available requires specialized biochemical microassay[36] and is unsuitable for conventional procedures.

These factors prompted us to investigate the value of histochemistry in detecting androgen binding sites in prostatic tissue specimens. In 1978 we reported development of a fluorescent ligand composed of testosterone linked by a hemisuccinate bridge to bovine serum albumin (BSA) which was then labeled with fluorescein isothiocyanate (FITC).[37] We used a conjugate with a ratio of steroid to BSA to label of 9:1:5. We later synthesized a similar conjugate using dihydrotestosterone (DHT), which gave the same staining pattern.

## II. METHODOLOGY FOR HISTOCHEMICAL ANDROGEN BINDING ASSAY

The methodology for the determination of androgen binding (AB) in tissue sections has been previously outlined.[38] Frozen tumor sections, 4 μm in thickness, were mounted on gelatin-coated slides to improve adherence and incubated with $7 \times 10^{-7}$ $M$ of ligand-conjugate for 2 hr at room temperature. The sections were rinsed with phosphate buffered saline (PBS), pH 7.1 to 7.4, postfixed in ethanol/acetone, and triple washed in PBS. Parallel sections were incubated with the same concentration of BSA-FITC unlinked to a steroid in order to monitor nonspecific binding of BSA. Competitive binding studies were also run in parallel with a molar excess of unlabeled DHT or antiandrogen. Specimens containing 10% or more of positively stained tumor cells were considered to be positive when processed sections were studied by appropriate incident light ultraviolet microscopy.

## III. SPECIFICITY STUDIES WITH FLUORESCENT ANDROGENS

The fluorescent androgens were tested on a wide variety of human and animal tissues and tissue culture cells. Fluorescence was only visible in preparations from organs known to contain AR by biochemical assay. When compared to the synthetic androgen R1881 commonly used as a ligand in biochemical AR assays, it was found that 240 nmol of conjugate was equivalent to 1 nmol R1881 in its displacement of radioactive R1881.[39] Upon reaction with the transplanted rat prostatic carcinoma Dunning R3327-H and R3327-A and human cell line DU 145,[40-42] the well-differentiated, slowly growing, hormone-sensitive, biochemically AR-positive R3327-H tumors displayed a high level of cytoplasmic and nuclear binding (Figure 1), whereas the rapidly growing, poorly differentiated, hormone-insensitive, biochemically AR-negative R3327-A and DU 145 tumors displayed a paucity of ligand binding. In addition, in fluorescent competitive binding studies with unlabeled androgens, other steroids, antisteroids, and synthetic ligands, the best inhibition was exhibited by the androgens and antiandrogens.

## IV. COMPARISON OF HISTOCHEMICAL AND BIOCHEMICAL ANDROGEN BINDING ASSAYS

Results of histochemical AB and biochemical AR analyses were compared in two series of cases. In the first series,[38] AR by dextran-coated charcoal assay (DCC) was performed by Dr. D. T. Zava in the laboratory of Dr. William McGuire, University of Texas Health Sciences Center, San Antonio, Tex. Results were available for comparison in 54 cases of benign and malignant prostatic disease. In the second series,[39] AB was correlated with AR by DCC performed by Hannah Rosenthal in the laboratory of Dr. A. Sandberg, Roswell Park Memorial Institute, Buffalo, N.Y. In the latter study, 77 prostate cancer specimens were analyzed. Criteria for biochemical AR positivity differed in the two series. In series I, specimens containing >7 fmol AR per milligram DNA were designated as positive, while in series II, tumors containing any measurable specific binding of R1881 were considered positive. The latter were subdivided into groups showing zero, trace <150, low 150 to 350, intermediate >350 to 550, high >550 to 950, and very high >950 fmol/g tissue for eventual comparison with semiquantified AB results.

Comparison of AB by histochemistry and AR by DCC in these 131 specimens is shown in Table 1. In series I, the presence or absence of AB and AR correlated in 89%, while there was concordance in 82% of the specimens studied in series II. Thus, there was overall agreement of results in 85% of the samples studied. A Fischer Exact Probability test applied to these data indicated that it was very unlikely that results were due to chance alone ($p$ <0.01). Several other comparisons could be made in series II. Cytosol and nuclear biochemical AR levels were measured separately and, thus, could be compared with the subcellular distribution of androgen observed microscopically (Table 2). In this comparison, there was agreement in 78% with a close association between methods as well as a high level of concordance ($p$ <0.0001, K = 0.673). Furthermore, the level of androgen bound was semiquantified as described in our chapter on methods of quantification and grouped for comparison with the quantified biochemical data (Table 3). Statistical analyses for agreement of equivalent or neighboring classifications again showed a significant association ($p$ <0.005, K = 0.342).

## V. CYTOPLASMIC VS. NUCLEAR ANDROGEN BINDING

The location of AB by histochemistry in nucleus and/or cytoplasm appeared to be primarily dependent upon the surgical technique utilized to obtain the sample. When specimens were

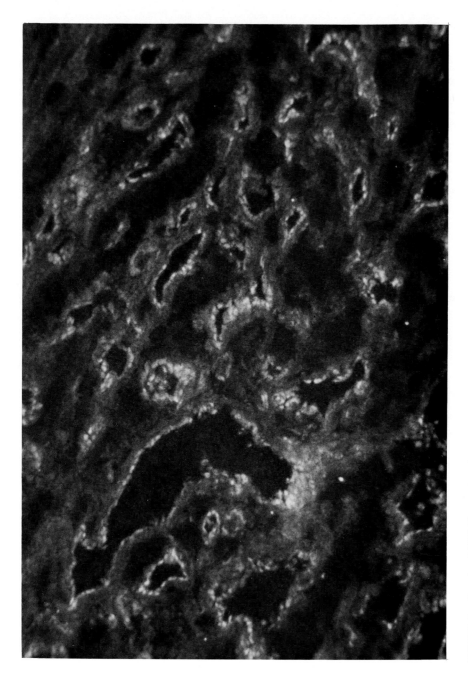

FIGURE 1. Dunning R3327-H transplanted rat adenocarcinoma demonstrating predominantly nuclear androgen binding in the epithelial cell component. Note absence of stromal staining. (Magnification $\times$ 100.)

**Table 1**
**COMPARISON OF ANDROGEN**
**BINDING BY HISTOCHEMISTRY AND**
**BIOCHEMICAL ANDROGEN**
**RECEPTOR IN PROSTATIC NEOPLASIA**

| Biochemical assay[a] | Histochemical assay[a] | | |
|---|---|---|---|
| | Positive | Negative | Total |
| Positive | 100 | 8 | 108 |
| Negative | 12 | 11 | 23 |
| Total | 112 | 19 | 131 |

[a]   See text for derivation of categories.

**Table 2**
**SUBCELLULAR ANDROGEN BINDING SITES: COMPARISON OF**
**HISTOCHEMISTRY WITH BIOCHEMISTRY**

| Biochemical assay | Histochemical assay | | | |
|---|---|---|---|---|
| | Cytoplasm | Nucleus | Cytoplasm and nucleus | None |
| Cytosol | 28 | 5 | 2 | 1 |
| Nuclear extract | 2 | 3 | 0 | 1 |
| Cytosol and nuclear extract | 0 | 0 | 21 | 1 |
| None | 1 | 3 | 0 | 5 |

**Table 3**
**SEMIQUANTITATIVE HISTOCHEMICAL ANDROGEN**
**BINDING IN PROSTATE CANCER. COMPARISON WITH**
**BIOCHEMICAL ANDROGEN RECEPTORS**

| Biochemical assay (fmol/g tissue) | Histochemical assay[a] | | |
|---|---|---|---|
| | Zero—trace | Low—intermediate | High—very high |
| Zero—trace (0—149) | 7 | 8 | 3 |
| Low—intermediate (150—550) | 6 | 11 | 3 |
| High—very high (>550) | 4 | 6 | 13 |

[a]   See chapter on "Methods of Quantification" for derivation of categories.

obtained by electrocautery, nuclear binding tended to predominate, whereas in specimens procured without the application of heat, nuclear binding was distinctly less commonly observed. In 103 specimens specifically analyzed for this phenomenon, nuclear binding predominated in 19 of 46 specimens (41%) secured by electrocautery, but was only seen in 1 of 57 specimens obtained without the use of heat. Conversely, cytoplasmic staining predominated in only 14 (30%) of electrocautery specimens, while it dominated in 77% of the specimens obtained by cold-knife or needle biopsy. Chi-square analysis showed that these observations were of statistical significance ($p < 0.0001$).

After having noted the above findings we asked our participating urologists to perform a needle biopsy on several patients with prostatic carcinoma about to undergo transurethral prostatic resection (TURP). In 7 of 11 cases there was a marked increase in nuclear AB in specimens obtained by TURP as compared to the needle biopsy specimens (Figures 2A and 2B). The mechanism underlying this change in binding locale may be related to heat-induced nuclear translocation of binding protein.

The stroma of specimens secured by TURP not infrequently also exhibited nuclear AB, whereas the stroma of samples obtained without the use of heat rarely showed any visible fluorescence above background. We believe that concentration of binding proteins in a small cellular structure such as the nucleus occurs after exposure to heat, whereas dissipation of binding sites in the cytoplasm of stromal cells otherwise prevents their detection. This increase in nuclear binding as a result of electrocautery, as well as exposure to 37°C in vitro, has also been observed by Nenci and colleagues.[43] Examples of nuclear and cytoplasmic epithelial androgen binding in prostatic carcinoma are shown in Figures 3 and 4. Stromal nuclear binding of androgen is illustrated in Figure 5.

## VI. CORRELATION OF HISTOCHEMICAL ANDROGEN BINDING ASSAY WITH CLINICAL RESPONSE TO ENDOCRINE THERAPY

At this writing we have examined prostate carcinoma specimens from 77 men treated by various forms of hormonal manipulation. Objective evaluation of therapeutic response was made according to the criteria outlined by the National Prostatic Cancer Project.[44]

In this group of men we classified the degree of androgen binding in the following way. Cases were considered as negative when less than 10% of the tumor cells were positive for AB. Cases were designated as borderline positive when 10 to 20% of the constituent malignant cells were stained, and as positive when more than 20% of tumor cells were fluorescent.

In 28 of the 77 cases, the only therapy employed was diethylstilbestrol (DES). Nineteen were positive for androgen binding. Eight responded, one evidenced a mixed response (regression of disease in some areas, progression in others), six had their disease process stabilized, while the remaining four failed, i.e., progressed. Five patients were borderline positive. One progressed, one was stabilized, and three had a successful response. Four patients were AB-negative. Two progressed and two became stable.

In 11 cases the primary therapy was orchiectomy. Nine were positive for androgen binding. Four responded and five were stabilized. One borderline positive and one negative case progressed.

Thirteen men were treated both by castration and with DES. Nine were positive for androgen binding. Six responded, one was stabilized, and two failed. Three patients with AB-negative tumors and one with a borderline-positive lesion progressed.

Flutamide was used to treat two patients. One AB-positive case failed. One negative patient became stabilized. Four others were treated by orchiectomy in combination with flutamide. Two were AB-positive. One responded and one failed. One was borderline positive and failed as did the remaining patient who was AB-negative.

Five men were already taking DES at the time of biopsy after which the dosage was increased. Three were positive for androgen binding. One patient responded, one was stabilized, while the other failed. One borderline positive and one negative case failed.

Two men initially were orchiectomized, but because of progressive disease were rebiopsied and then started on DES. Both had negative assays and both failed. Three others had been orchiectomized and were taking DES initially but had failed and required additional surgery, after which the DES dosage was increased. Two were AB-positive. One responded while the other was stabilized. The third patient had a negative assay and continued to progress.

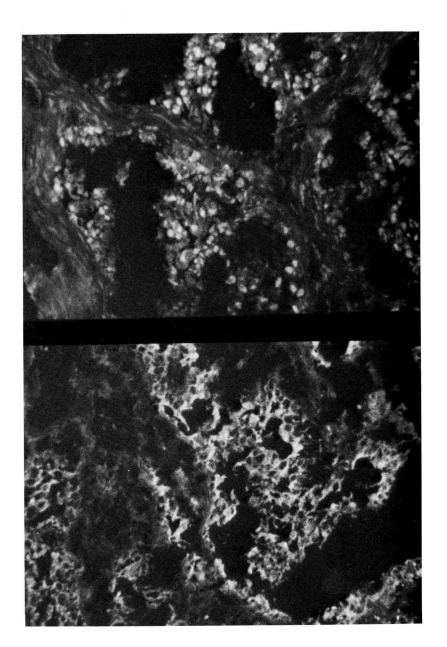

FIGURE 2. (A, left) Prostatic adenocarcinoma specimen obtained by needle biopsy showing cytoplasmic uptake of androgen ligand-conjugate. Heterogeneity of binding is evident. (Magnification × 100.) (B, right) Electroresected sample from the same patient exhibiting nuclear androgen binding primarily. Heterogeneity is still apparent. (Magnification × 100.)

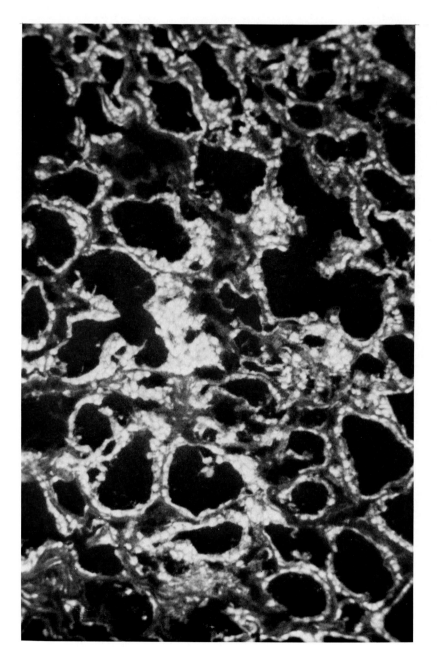

FIGURE 3.   Well-differentiated prostatic adenocarcinoma exhibiting nuclear uptake of androgen ligand. Considerable binding heterogeneity is present. Specimen was obtained by TURP. (Magnification × 100.)

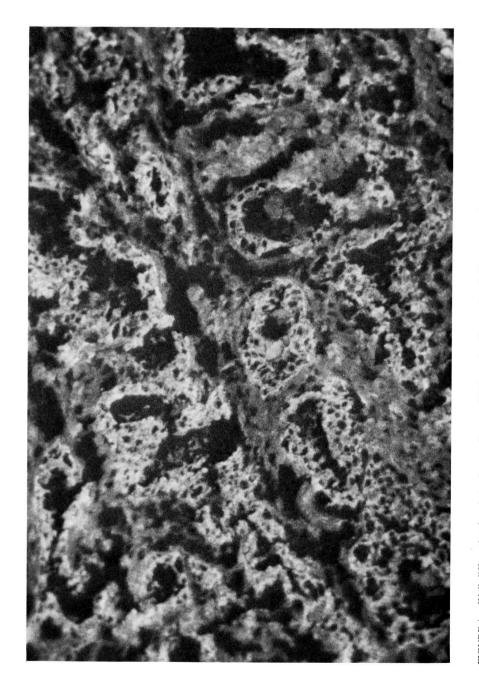

FIGURE 4.    Well-differentiated prostate adenocarcinoma exhibiting primarily cytoplasmic fluorescence after exposure to androgen ligand-conjugate. Note the binding heterogeneity which is present. Specimen obtained by retropubic prostatectomy with a cold knife. (Magnification $\times$ 100.)

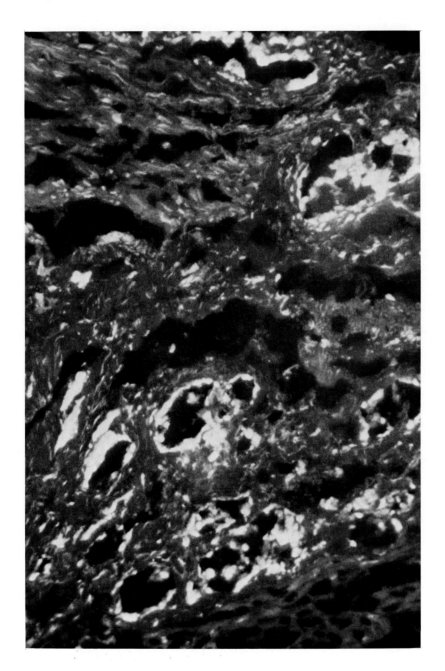

**FIGURE 5.**    Electroresected sample of prostatic adenocarcinoma exhibiting stromal as well as tumor cell androgen ligand uptake.  (Magnification × 100.)

**Table 4**
### HISTOCHEMICAL ANDROGEN BINDING ASSAY: RELATIONSHIP TO ENDOCRINE RESPONSE IN PROSTATE CANCER

| Assay results[a] | Responded | Stable | Failed | Total |
|---|---|---|---|---|
| Positive | 24 | 15 | 11 | 50 |
| Borderline positive | 3 | 1 | 5 | 9 |
| Negative | 0 | 3 | 15 | 18 |
| Total | 27 | 19 | 31 | 77 |

[a]  See text for criteria of positivity and negativity.

Seven men were on DES and failing. They were then rebiopsied and castrated. Five were AB-positive. Two responded, one was stabilized, and two failed. Two AB-negative cases also failed. Another two men had failed orchiectomy, were rebiopsied, found to be AB-negative, and continued to fail without any additional treatment.

Table 4 summarizes the results of this ongoing study. It can be seen that of the 18 negative cases, 15 failed to respond to endocrine therapy. The predictive value of a negative AB assay for failure was, thus, 83%. On the other hand, of the 50 AB-positive men, a total of 39 either responded or had their disease stabilized. The predictive value of a positive assay was, therefore, 78%. The sensitivity of the AB assay, i.e., the number of responders or stabilized patients with a positive assay, was 93%. The specificity, i. e., the number of failures with a negative assay, was 48%. There are too few patients in the borderline-positive category to warrant a definitive statement. In this low positive group were nine cases. Five failed, one was stabilized, and three responded. Statistical evaluation of the observed difference in the percentage of AB-positive and AB-negative patients failing therapy, i. e., 27% vs. 83% showed that the probability that this was due to chance alone was remote ($p$ <0.001) by chi-square analysis.

## VII. ESTROGEN BINDING IN PROSTATIC CARCINOMA

ER has been detected in prostatic tissues by several investigators,[10,31,38,45] but the significance and relationship to endocrine response in prostate cancer is unknown.

In our laboratory, we have performed estrogen binding (EB) studies using 17-beta-estradiol-hemisuccinyl-BSA-FITC (17-FE). In 62 cases of prostatic cancer we correlated EB with the outcome of hormonal therapy. The predictive value of a positive assay for response was 72%, while the predictive value of a negative assay for failure was 70%. Thus, EB does not appear to be as useful a marker for endocrine response as AB. There are insufficient numbers of cases to determine the effectiveness of combined EB and AB assays in prognostication since most of our AB-positive cases were also positive for EB. There are too few AB-positive, EB-negative, or AB-negative, EB-positive cases to currently evaluate.

In a study utilizing estradiol-3-dansylate as a fluorescent histochemical probe, Van Dalen[46] reported that about 50% of transperineal biopsies of prostate cancer showed cytoplasmic staining. He noted a lower level of positivity in tissue obtained from distant metastases and suggested that aggressive lesions might be more likely to be low in EB. Our results show little difference in the percentage of specimens positive for AB/EB in grade 1 vs. grade 5 tumors, or in specimens from patients with stage IA compared to D2 disease.[39] However, in those few specimens we have studied from prostatic carcinoma metastases, 60% were borderline positive or negative compared to 35% of primary tumors. This situation may be analogous to breast cancer metastases where concordance between ER levels in the primary neoplasm and metastases was found in only 46%.[47]

## VIII. OTHER HISTOCHEMICAL STUDIES OF STEROID BINDING IN THE PROSTATE

There exists, to our knowledge, only three other histochemical studies designed to detect steroid binding in prostatic tissue. Naito et al.,[48] using a labeled derivative of R1881 to study prostate hyperplasia, found good concordance with biochemical AR levels. However, since R1881 may also bind to progesterone receptor (PgR),[12] binding to AR could not clearly be distinguished from binding to PgR. These workers commented upon the lack of nuclear and stromal staining. This probably was due to their specimens being obtained by retropubic prostatectomy with a cold knife.

In a study of six human prostatic carcinoma specimens and three from men with benign hyperplasia together with a number of rat prostates, Lammel et al.,[49] using a fluoresceinated DHT derivative, encountered a number of ambiguities and concluded that their ligand was not suitable for appropriate demonstration of AR. On the other hand, Matsumura et al.,[50] using labeled R1881 as the binding ligand, studied 55 samples of prostate cancer. They found that well-differentiated and moderately differentiated cancers were significantly more likely to be positive. They also noted that patients who had relapsed after endocrine therapy were more likely to have a negative assay. Of greater importance, 100% of 34 patients with positive staining responded to endocrine treatment, while 50% of their negative cases failed.

## IX. STUDIES OF PROSTATIC CARCINOMA WITH MONOCLONAL ANTIBODIES TO ESTROGEN RECEPTOR

Utilizing the estrogen receptor immunocytochemical assay (ERICA) of Greene et al.,[51-53] we have studied over 100 specimens of prostatic carcinoma and at this time have encountered only one specimen which showed some focal positive staining. Greene and colleagues have not seen positive staining in prostate tissue in a smaller number of cases.[54] Ekman and colleagues also did not observe any positive staining.[55] It, therefore, appears that ERICA cannot be used to assess ER in prostatic tissue. Possibly, prostatic ER differs antigenically. It is also possible that the level of ER in prostate cells is below the limits of detectability with ERICA. The lack of positive staining is not related to the manner of specimen procurement. Specimens secured by cold knife, by needle, or TURP were all equally negative.

## X. MULTIPLICITY OF ESTROGEN BINDING SITES IN PROSTATIC CARCINOMA

In our chapter on breast cancer we have detailed the biochemical and histochemical evidence for a multiplicity of estrogen binding sites. There is now similar evidence that this is also the case in prostatic tissues. In a recent study, Ekman et al.[55] described the presence of type II ER in samples of benign and malignant prostate.

Intrigued by our inability to detect ER in prostate utilizing ERICA and by our findings in breast cancer, we investigated 79 specimens of prostatic adenocarcinoma with 17-FE and compared results with EB using 17-beta-estradiol-6-$O$-carboxymethyloxime-BSA-FITC (6-FE) by the method of Lee.[56] Any specimen with at least 10% tumor cells exhibiting a +1 fluorescent intensity was considered as positive. Results are shown in Tables 5 and 6.

Assay results were in essential agreement as to positivity or negativity in 73%. Forty-eight specimens were positive with both 17-FE and 6-FE while ten were negative with both

**Table 5**
**COMPARISON OF**
**HISTOCHEMICAL ESTROGEN**
**BINDING ASSAYS USING 6-FE**
**AND 17-FE IN PROSTATE**
**CANCER**

|         | 6-FE + | 6-FE − | Total |
|---------|--------|--------|-------|
| 17-FE + | 48     | 16     | 64    |
| 17-FE − | 5      | 10     | 15    |
| Total   | 53     | 26     | 79    |

**Table 6**
**COMPARISON OF SUBCELLULAR ESTROGEN**
**BINDING WITH 6-FE AND 17-FE IN**
**ESTROGEN BINDING-POSITIVE PROSTATIC**
**CARCINOMAS**

| 17-FE       | 6-FE        |         |           |       |
|-------------|-------------|---------|-----------|-------|
|             | Cytoplasmic | Nuclear | Nucleolar | Total |
| Cytoplasmic | 30          | 1       | 0         | 31    |
| Nuclear     | 5           | 11      | 1         | 17    |
| Nucleolar   | 0           | 0       | 0         | 0     |
| Total       | 35          | 12      | 1         | 48    |

conjugates. There were 16 specimens that were 17-FE-positive and 6-FE-negative and 5 that were 17-FE-negative and 6-FE-positive. Considerable differences in staining pattern were also noted. Since 6-FE has more moles of FITC per mole BSA than does 17-FE, it would be expected that staining with 6-FE would be more intense as is true for breast cancer. However, in 11 cases of prostate cancer, staining with 17-FE was considerably brighter than with 6-FE, and in only 17 cases was staining with 6-FE of greater intensity. In the remaining cases, staining was felt to be of about equal magnitude.

The subcellular localization of staining with both 17-FE and 6-FE was cytoplasmic in 30 specimens and nuclear in 11. However, five samples showed nuclear 17-FE and cytoplasmic 6-FE and one nuclear 6-FE and cytoplasmic 17-FE. Another sample contained nuclear 17-FE and nucleolar 6-FE. In several specimens it was quite apparent that different cell populations bound each ligand.

In all of the above cases, ERICA was negative. These results clearly show that what is recognized by ERICA is different to what is detected by the ligand-conjugates and also suggests that 6-FE and 17-FE recognize separate but associated estrogen binding sites in prostate cancer (putative type II sites) as well as in breast cancer.

## XI. ADVANTAGES OF HISTOCHEMICAL STEROID BINDING ASSAYS IN PROSTATIC CARCINOMA

During our investigations of steroid binding in prostatic tissue some of the advantages of a histochemical technique became obvious. Several specimens were encountered where benign and malignant cells were admixed. When both were positive or both negative for

AB, no harm would have resulted from a positive or negative biochemical AR. On the other hand, we have seen three specimens where only the benign component was AB-positive while the majority of cancer cells were AB-negative. In all three cases, biochemical AR was positive suggesting that the patient might successfully respond to hormonal manipulation. In actuality, all three patients progressed on hormonal therapy as was anticipated from the histochemical results.

We have had the opportunity to study several unusual prostatic malignancies. One such specimen was a leiomyosarcoma of the prostate that was AB-negative. We also have examined two prostatic carcinosarcomas. In one, both sarcomatous and carcinomatous elements were AB-negative. However, while the sarcomatous elements were EB-negative, the epithelial component was EB-positive. In the second case, both epithelial and sarcomatous elements were both EB- and AB-positive.

Heterogeneity of steroid binding is commonly encountered in prostate cancer and may be assessed histochemically by estimating the numbers of cells showing various levels of fluorescent intensity. In theory, heterogeneity of steroid binding should be of great significance. It is only reasonable to anticipate that length of response to endocrine therapy should correlate with the degree of observed heterogeneity. Hypothetically, the larger the proportion of negative and borderline-positive cells, the shorter the interval of hormone response. At this time we do not possess sufficient data to test this hypothesis. In theory, also, if a patient who had previously responded to hormonal treatment begins to fail, this should be associated with a proliferation of cells capable of autonomous growth. This should be manifested histochemically by an increased number of negative cells. Again, however, we do not yet possess enough data to support or refute this hypothesis. However, it should be noted that in the clinical correlative study described previously were 19 men who had already been subjected to hormonal manipulation at the time of AB assay. In this small group there were nine (47%) with negative or borderline assays compared to 31% in untreated cases.

Another advantage of the histochemical method relates to the high proportion of specimens submitted for steroid binding assay which fail to contain tumor upon light microscopic examination. In this study 9.6% of all specimens submitted did not contain tumor. It is apparent that all specimens submitted for biochemical steroid receptor assays should be first examined histologically to verify the presence of tumor, otherwise results would be spurious and misleading in a significant number of cases. The reason for the large number of specimens without tumor is associated with the difficulty in recognition of tumor by gross examination of prostatic samples.

## XII. ANDROGEN BINDING IN PROSTATIC DISEASE OTHER THAN CARCINOMA

A total of 631 specimens from patients with benign prostatic hyperplasia (BPH) were analyzed for AB and EB: 430 (68%) were AB-positive, EB-positive, 28 (5%) were AB-positive, EB-negative, 27 (4%) were AB-negative, EB-positive, and 103 (16%) were EB-negative and AB-negative. Forty-three specimens were either too severely damaged by electrocautery or failed to contain any glandular elements, and could not, therefore, be assayed.

Heterogeneity of binding was not as common a feature in BPH as in cancer but was occasionally noted on a regional basis. Thus, if any one gland were positive, nearly all the cells comprising the gland were positive. On the other hand, several positive glands might be observed in one area of the tissue while another area might contain several negative glands.

The large number of specimens analyzed permitted several observations to be made. Seven specimens were prostate infiltrated by transitional cell carcinoma of the urinary bladder.

These urothelial carcinomas were all AB/EB-negative. The presence of large numbers of inflammatory cells as in chronic prostatitis were associated with poor ligand uptake. Almost half (40%) of such specimens were negative. Two specimens of granulomatous prostatitis were AB/EB-negative. As might be expected, infarction of the prostate was also associated with a high degree of negativity; 60% of infarcted specimens exhibited a low level of steroid binding. Squamous metaplasia of prostate glands was also associated with a low level of binding.

The type of surgical procedure used to obtain the tissue specimen influenced location of steroid in nucleus or cytoplasm as in prostate cancer. Specimens obtained by TURP showed a much higher proportion of nuclear binding than did those secured without the use of a heating current and, also, had a tendency to be low or poor steroid binders. Apparently, excessive heat can destroy the tissue steroid binding capability entirely. In 32 cases a pre-TURP needle biopsy and a TURP specimen were available for study. In 20 (62%) cytoplasmic staining predominated in the needle biopsy, whereas the corresponding TURP specimen primarily exhibited nuclear binding. In the remaining 28% of specimens, the needle biopsy was positive while the TURP sample was negative. A decrease in AR in TURP specimens has also been detected by biochemical assay.[57,58]

## XIII. DETECTION OF ENDOGENOUS STEROID BOUND IN VIVO

Since it might be anticipated that receptor bound to steroid in vivo would not be available for binding to ligand, we initially felt that it was important to develop a technique for the detection of endogenous-bound hormone. This was accomplished by a standard indirect immunofluorescence assay (IF). Fixed, frozen tissue sections were washed in buffer and incubated with rabbit antiserum to estradiol and testosterone in parallel. After rewashing the tissue was exposed to fluoresceinated goat-anti-rabbit immunoglobulin. A 60-min buffer wash completed the procedure. As a control, positive tissues were restudied with specifically absorbed antiserum.

We looked for in vivo bound steroid in 103 prostatic carcinoma specimens and detected androgen in 12% and estrogen in 11%. A significantly larger proportion of patients in the younger age groups were found to be positive. However, in no instance could it be shown that the presence of endogenous steroid interfered with binding of the steroid ligand-conjugates, and in the case of androgens, with the biochemical detection of AR. It appeared that not all the available binding sites were bound and that a significant number were available for binding of ligand. Of interest it may be noted that a not dissimilar finding regarding in vivo bound steroid has been reported in the rat prostate cancer model.[41] As a consequence of this study we felt that abandonment of endogenous steroid detection as a routine procedure was warranted in these studies.

## XIV. RELATIONSHIP BETWEEN PROSTATIC ACID PHOSPHATASE AND ANDROGEN BINDING BY HISTOCHEMISTRY

In order to determine if there was any relationship between the presence of prostatic acid phosphatase (PAP) and androgen binding, we processed 81 specimens of prostatic carcinoma in parallel for both of these tumor markers. For PAP detection, an IF procedure was used employing a 1:200 dilution of a potent, polyclonal antiserum, made in goat and generously donated by Dr. Chu Ming of the Roswell Park Memorial Institute. Ethanol-fixed frozen sections were reacted wtih the PAP antiserum and then labeled with fluoresceinated rabbit-anti-goat immunoglobulin.

In this series of cases, 33 specimens (41%) were PAP+ as well as positive for androgen binding and an equal number were PAP+ and negative for androgen. Eight (10%) were

PAP— and positive for androgen binding while the remaining 7 (9%) were negative for both PAP and androgen. Furthermore, even in those specimens which were positive for both PAP and androgen, it could be seen that different cell populations were labeled. We, therefore, concluded that no relationship existed between these tumor markers.

## XV. THE NATURE OF THE BINDING REVEALED BY HISTOCHEMICAL STEROID BINDING ASSAYS IN PROSTATE

In our chapter on steroid binding in breast cancer we have detailed our investigations into the nature of the binding revealed by histochemical methods in that organ. We concluded that for estrogen, and probably for progesterone, there exists a multiplicity of binding sites, and that currently it was felt that the BSA steroid conjugates are quite likely binding to the lower affinity receptor sites, i.e., type II. However, certain experimental evidence, in particular the ability of these methods to demonstrate apparent nuclear translocation, was not consistent with this conclusion. At this time, therefore, it is best not to make any unequivocal judgements.

Only lately have we begun to accumulate data indicating that patients who are positive for androgen binding with both histochemical and biochemical assays do better on endocrine therapy than patients positive with only one method. Recently received biochemical values from Dr. Sidney Shain, Southwest Foundation for Research and Education, San Antonio, Tex. has enabled the evaluation of 46 men where results of both assay systems are known. In this group, the positive predictive value of the histochemical assay was 78% and the negative predictive value 100%. Specificity was 40% and sensitivity 100%. For the biochemical assay, positive and negative predictive values were both 78%. Specificity = 47% and sensitivity = 94%. However, when both assay results were combined, the positive predictive value rose to 86% while the negative predictive value was 91%. Sensitivity was 97% and specificity 67% ($p < 0.05$). These preliminary results suggest that histochemical and biochemical androgen binding assays recognize separate but closely related sites, and that there is a degree of cooperativity between these sites. More cases must be studied before the validity of these findings can be established.

## ACKNOWLEDGMENTS

Ms. Evelyn Rainford and Ms. Ethel Jones provided valued technical expertise. Dr. E. Gaetjens supplied the labeled androgen and estrogen (17-FE) ligand-conjugates. We thank Zeus Scientific, Inc. for the gift of 6-FE, Roussel UCLAF for R1881 (methyltrienolone), Schering AG for cyproterone acetate, and Schering Corp. for Flutamide. Merck Sharp & Dohme donated the antiandrogen MK 316.

We are indebted to the following urologists for providing tissue specimens and allowing access to the clinical records of their cases: Drs. H. Kim and D. S. Kim, Brookdale Hospital Center, Dr. J. Abrahams, Brooklyn Veterans Administration Hospital, Dr. G. Wise, Maimonides Medical Center, Dr. W. F. Whitmore, Jr. and Dr. H. Herr, Memorial Sloan-Kettering Cancer Center.

# REFERENCES

1. **Huggins, C. and Hodges, C.,** Studies on prostatic cancer. I. The effect of castration, of estrogen and of androgen injection on serum phosphatases in metastatic carcinoma of the prostate, *Cancer Res.,* 1, 293, 1941.
2. Veterans Administration Cooperative Urological Research Group, Carcinoma of the prostate: treatment comparison, *J. Urol.,* 98, 516, 1967.
3. Veterans Administration Cooperative Urological Research Group, Factors in the prognosis of carcinoma of the prostate, a cooperative study, *Surg. Gynecol. Obstet.,* 124, 1011, 1967.
4. **Hansson, V., Tveter, K. J., Attramadal, A., and Torgerson, O.,** Androgen receptors in human nodular prostatic hyperplasia, *Acta Endocrinol.,* 68, 79, 1971.
5. **Geller, J., Cantor, T., and Albert, J.,** Evidence for a specific dihydrotestosterone binding cytosol receptor in human prostate, *J. Clin. Endocrinol. Metab.,* 41, 854, 1975.
6. **Cowan, R. A., Cowan, S. K., and Grant, J. K.,** The specificity of 5α-dihydrotestosterone binding in human prostate cytosol preparations, *Biochem. Soc. Trans.,* 3, 537, 1975.
7. **Rosen, V., Jung, I., Baulieu, E.-E., and Robel, P.,** Androgen-binding proteins in human benign prostatic hypertrophy, *J. Clin. Endocrinol. Metab.,* 41, 761, 1975.
8. **Menon, M., Tananis, C. E., McLaughlin, M. G., and Walsh, P.,** Androgen receptors in human prostate: a review, *Cancer Treat. Rep.,* 61, 265, 1977.
9. **Mainwaring, W. I. P. and Milroy, E. J. G.,** Characterization of the specific androgen receptors in the human prostate gland, *J. Endocrinol.,* 57, 371, 1973.
10. **Wagner, R. K., Schulze, K. H., and Jungblut, P. W.,** Estrogen and androgen receptor in human prostate and prostate tumor tissue, *Acta Endocrinol.,* 193 (Suppl.), 52, 1975.
11. **Asselin, J., Labrie, F., Gourdeau, Y., Bonne, C., and Raynaud, J.-P,** Binding of ($^3$H) Methyltrienolone (R1881) in rat prostate and human benign prostatic hypertrophy (BPH), *Steroids,* 28, 449, 1976.
12. **Snochowski, M., Pousette, A., Ekman, P., Bression, D., Andersson, L., Högberg, B., and Gustafsson, J.-A,** Characterization and measurement of the androgen receptor in human benign prostatic hyperplasia and prostate carcinoma, *J. Clin. Endocrinol. Metab.,* 45, 920, 1977.
13. **Mobbs, B. G., Johnson, I. E., Connolly, J. G., and Clark, A. F.,** Evaluation of the use of cyproterone acetate competition to distinguish between high affinity binding of ($^3$H) dihydrotestosterone to human prostate cytosol receptors and to sex steroid hormone binding globulins, *J. Steroid Biochem.,* 8, 943, 1977.
14. **Hawkins, H. F., Nijs, M., and Brassine, C.,** Steroid receptors in the human prostate. Detection of tissue specific androgen binding in prostate cancer, *Clin. Chem.,* 77, 101, 1978.
15. **Sirett, D. and Grant, J. K.,** Androgen binding in cytosols and nuclei of human benign hyperplastic prostatic tissue, *J. Endocrinol.,* 77, 101, 1978.
16. **Menon, M., Tananis, C. E., McLaughlin, M. G., Lippmann, M. E., and Walsh, P. C.,** The measurement of androgen receptors in human prostatic tissue utilizing sucrose density centrifugation and a protamine precipitation assay, *J. Urol.,* 117, 309, 1977.
17. **Kodama, T., Honda, S., and Shimazaki, J.,** Androphilic proteins in cytosols of benign prostatic hypertrophy, *Endocrinol. Jpn.,* 24, 565, 1977.
18. **Mobbs, B. J., Johnson, I. E., Connolly, J. G., and Clark, A. F.,** Androgen receptor assay in human benign and malignant tumor cytosol using protamine sulphate precipitation, *J. Steroid Biochem.,* 9, 289, 1978.
19. **Krieg, M., Bartsch, W., Becker, H., and Voigt, K. D.,** Quantification of androgen binding, androgen tissue levels and sex hormone binding globulin in prostate, muscle and plasma of patients with benign prostatic hypertrophy, *Acta Endocrinol.,* 86, 200, 1977.
20. **Krieg, M., Grobe, I., Voigt, K. D., Altenahr, E., and Klosterhalfen, H.,** Human prostatic carcinoma: significant difference in its androgen binding and metabolism compared to the human benign prostatic hypertrophy, *Acta Endocrinol.,* 88, 397, 1978.
21. **Shain, S. A., Boessel, R. W., Lamm, D. L., and Radwin, H. M.,** Characterization of unoccupied (R) and occupied (RA) androgen binding components of the hyperplastic human prostate, *Steroids,* 31, 541, 1978.
22. **Ghanadian, R., Auf, G., Chaloner, P. J., and Chisholm, G. D.,** The use of methyltrienolone in the measurement of the free and bound cytoplasmic receptors for dihydrotestosterone in benign hypertrophied human prostate, *J. Steroid Biochem.,* 9, 325, 1978.
23. **Symes, E. K., Milroy, E. J. G., and Mainwaring, W. I. P.,** The nuclear uptake of androgen by human benign prostate *in vitro:* action of antiandrogens, *J. Urol.,* 120, 180, 1978.
24. **Bonne, C. and Raynaud, J.-P.,** Methyltrienolone, a specific ligand for cellular androgen receptors, *Steroids,* 26, 227, 1975.
25. **de Voogt, H. J. and Linjan, P.,** Steroid receptors in human prostatic cancer. A preliminary evaluation, *Urol. Res.,* 6, 151, 1978.

26. **Ekman, P., Snochowski, M., Dahlberg, E., and Gustaffson, J.-A.,** Steroid receptors in metastatic carcinoma of the human prostate, *Eur. J. Cancer,* 15, 257, 1979.

27. **Ekman, P., Snochowski, M., Zetterberg, A., Högberg, B., and Gustaffson, J.-A.,** Steroid receptor content in human prostatic carcinoma and response to endocrine therapy, *Cancer,* 44, 1173, 1979.

28. **Geller, J., Albert, J., and Loza, D.,** Steroid levels in cancer of the prostate-markers of tumour differentiation and adequacy of anti-androgen therapy, *J. Steroid Biochem.,* 11, 631, 1979.

29. **Gustaffson, J.-A., Ekman, P., Snochowski, M., Zetterberg, A., Pousette, A., and Högberg, B.,** Correlation between clinical response to hormone therapy and steroid receptor content in prostatic cancer, *Cancer Res.,* 38, 4345, 1978.

30. **Mobbs, B. G., Johnson, I. E., and Connolly, J. G.,** Protamine sulfate precipitation of androgen receptors in cytosols of human benign and malignant prostate tumors, in *Prostate Cancer and Hormone Receptors,* Murphy, G. P. and Sandberg, A. A. Eds., Alan R. Liss, New York, 1979, 13.

31. **Sidh, S. M., Young, J. D., Karmi, S. A., and Bashirelahi, N.,** Adenocarcinoma of the prostate: role of 17β-estradiol and 5 α-dihydrotestosterone binding proteins, *Urology,* 13, 597, 1979.

32. **Martelli, A., Soli, M., Bercovich, E., Prodi, G., Grilli, S., DeGiovanni, C., and Galli, M. C.,** Correlation between clinical response to antiandrogen therapy and occurrence of receptors in human prostatic cancer, *Urology,* 16, 245, 1980.

33. **Ghanadian, R., Auf, G., Williams, G., and Richards, B.,** Predicting the response of prostatic carcinoma to endocrine therapy, *Lancet,* 2, 1418, 1981.

34. **Concolino, G., Marocchi, A., Margiotta, G., Conti, C., DeSilverio, F., Tenaglia, R., Ferraro, F., and Bracci, U.,** Steroid receptors and hormone responsiveness of human prostatic carcinoma, *Prostate,* 3, 475, 1982.

35. **Mainwaring, W. I. P.,** The relevance of studies on androgen action to prostatic cancer, in *Steroid Hormone Action and Cancer,* Menon, K. M. J. and Reel, J. R., Eds., Plenum Press, New York, 1975, 152.

36. **Trachtenberg, J., Hicks, L. L., and Walsh, P. C.,** Methods for the determination of androgen receptor content in human prostatic tissue, *Invest. Urol.,* 18, 349, 1981.

37. **Pertschuk, L. P., Zava, D. T., Gaetjens, E., Macchia, R. J., Brigati, D. J., and Kim, D. S.,** Detection of androgen and estrogen receptors in human prostatic carcinoma and hyperplasia by fluorescence microscopy, *Res. Commun. Chem. Pathol. Pharmacol.,* 22, 427, 1978.

38. **Pertschuk, L. P., Zava, D. T., Tobin, E. H., Brigati, D. J., Gaetjens, E., Macchia, R. J., Wise, G. J., Wax, H. S., and Kim, D. S.,** Histochemical detection of steroid hormone receptors in the human prostate, in *Prostate Cancer and Hormone Receptors,* Murphy, G. P. and Sandberg, A. A., Eds., Alan R. Liss, New York, 1979, 113.

39. **Pertschuk, L. P., Rosenthal, H. E., Macchia, R. J., Eisenberg, K. B., Feldman, J. G., Wax, S. H., Kim, D. S., Whitmore, W. F., Jr., Abrahams, J. I., Gaetjens, E., Wise, G. J., Herr, H. W., Karr, J. P., Murphy, G. P., and Sandberg, A. A.,** Correlation of histochemical and biochemical analyses of androgen binding in prostatic cancer: relation to therapeutic response, *Cancer,* 49, 984, 1982.

40. **Markland, F. S., Jr. and Lee, L.,** Characterization and comparison of the estrogen and androgen receptors from the R-3327 rat prostatic adenocarcinoma, *J. Steroid Biochem.,* 10, 13, 1979.

41. **Isaacs, J. T., Heston, W. D. W., Weissman, R. M., and Coffey, D. S.,** Animal models of the hormone-sensitive and -insensitive prostatic adenocarcinomas Dunning R-3327-H, R-3327-HI and R-3327-AT, *Cancer Res.,* 38, 4353, 1978.

42. **Stone, K. R., Mickey, D. D., Wunderli, H., Mickey, G. H., and Paulson, D. F.,** Isolation of a human prostate carcinoma cell line (DU 145), *Int. J. Cancer,* 21, 274, 1978.

43. **Nenci, I., Fabris, G., Mazzola, A., Bagni, A., Poli, G., and Marchetti, E.,** personal communication, 1983.

44. **Schmidt, J. D., Johnson, D. E., Scott, W. W., Gibbons, R. P., Prout, G. R., Jr., and Murphy, G. P.,** Chemotherapy of advanced prostatic cancer, evaluation of response parameters, *Urology,* 7, 602, 1976.

45. **Murphy, J. B., Emmott, R. C., Hicks, L. L., and Walsh, P. C.,** Estrogen receptors in the human prostate, seminal vesicles, epididymis, testis and genital skin: a marker for estrogen responsive tissues?, *J. Clin. Endocrinol. Metab.,* 50, 938, 1980.

46. **Van Dalen, J. P. R.,** Estradiol-3-dansylate used as a fluorescent histochemical stain, a possible prognostic aid for nondisseminating prostatic carcinoma, *J. Surg. Oncol.,* 17, 373, 1978.

47. **Holdaway, I. M. and Bowditch, J. V.,** Variation in receptor status between primary and metastatic breast cancer, *Cancer,* 52, 479, 1983.

48. **Naito, H., Ito, H., Wakisaka, M., Kambegawa, A., and Shimazaki, J.,** Histochemical observation of R1881 binding protein in human benign prostatic hypertrophy, *Invest. Urol.,* 18, 337, 1981.

49. **Lammel, A., Krieg, M., and Klotzi, G.,** Are fluorescein-conjugated androgens appropriate for a histochemical detection of prostatic androgen receptors?, *Prostate,* 4, 271, 1982.

50. **Matsumura, T., Naito, H., Yamaguchi, K., Ito, H., Matsuzaki, O., Kambegawar, A., and Shimazaki, J.,** Histochemical observation of R1881-binding protein in human prostatic cancer, *Urol. Invest.,* 38, 25, 1983.

51. **King, W. J., Jensen, E. V., Miller, L., and Greene, G. L.,** Immunocytochemical demonstration of estrogen receptor in frozen sections of human breast tumors with monoclonal anti-receptor antibodies, *Endocrinol. Suppl.,* 110, 258, 1982.

52. **Press, M. F., King, W., and Greene, G.,** Immunocytochemical localization of estrogen receptors in the human endometrium using a monoclonal antibody against human estrogen receptor, *Fed. Proc.,* 42, 1178, 1983.

53. **Pertschuk, L. P., Eisenberg, K. B., Carter, A. C., and Dayan, S. A.,** Estrogen receptor immunocytochemical assay with monoclonal antibodies. Correlation with biochemical assay in 103 cases and with clinical response to endocrine therapy in 32 cases, *Breast Cancer Res. Treat.,* 3, 304, 1983.

54. **Greene, G. L.,** personal communication, 1983.

55. **Ekman, P., Barrack, E. R., Greene, G. L., Jensen, E. V., and Walsh, P. C.,** Estrogen receptors in human prostate: evidence for multiple binding sites, *J. Clin. Endocrinol. Metab.,* 52, 166, 1983.

56. **Lee, S. H.,** Hydrophilic macromolecules of steroid derivatives for the detection of cancer cell receptors, *Cancer,* 46, 2825, 1980.

57. **Kitano, T., Usui, T., Yasukawa, A., Nakahara, M., Nihira, H., and Miyachi, Y.,** Androgen receptor in electroresected and cold punch-resected specimens, *Urology,* 21, 119, 1983.

58. **Albert, J., Geller, J., and Nachtsheim, D. A.,** The type of current frequency used in transurethral resection of prostate (TURP) affects the androgen receptor, *Prostate,* 3, 221, 1982.

Chapter 8

# BINDING OF LABELED ESTROGEN-ALBUMIN CONJUGATES IN BREAST CANCER

**J. van Marle, J.P.A. Baak, C.J.L.M. Meijer, and J. Lindeman**

## TABLE OF CONTENTS

I.      Introduction ........................................................................ 114

II.     Specificity of the Interaction between O-BSA-FITC Complex and Thin Sections of
        Mammary Tumors ............................................................... 115

III.    Correlation between Morphological Features of the Mammary Tumors and the
        Presence of Estrogen Receptors Assayed Biochemically ...................... 121
        A.      Methodology ....................................................... 122
        B.      Results ............................................................ 122
        C.      Comments .......................................................... 123

IV.     Correlation between Histochemical Method and Biochemical Assay ............ 124
        A.      Technical Details .................................................. 125
        B.      Criteria for the Interpretation of Results of Histochemical Assay ........ 126
        C.      Results and Concluding Remarks .................................... 126

References ................................................................................ 129

## I. INTRODUCTION

It was Lee[1] who was the first to use an estrogen-bovine serum albumin fluorescein isothiocyanate (O-BSA-FITC) complex in order to demonstrate estrogen binding sites in thin sections of mammary tumors. Synthesis of this O-BSA-FITC complex is relatively simple. This new method had the advantage over autoradiographic methods,[2] viz., with respect to technical simplicity and speed. In contrast to immunological methods,[3] the advantage of Lee's method is that no complicated purifications of antigen and antibodies are necessary and, besides, no animals have to be sensitized against either the estrogen receptor proper or estradiol. In his first publication Lee interpreted the fluorescence observed without any restrictions as proof of the presence of biochemically defined estrogen receptors. He did not specify the term receptor, but he implied its identity with the biochemically defined type I estrogen receptor.

Lee's method[1] was followed rapidly by the appearance of a number of publications[4-15] in which the distribution of the fluorescence in the sections and its association with certain cell types and histological properties of the mammary tumors were not studied as much as the correlation of the semiquantitatively estimated fluorescence with the biochemically determined amount of type I estrogen receptors.[4-9,13,15]

Some authors claim a close correlation,[4,6,8,9,15] but others did not find a correlation.[5,7,12,16]

It is surprising that only little attention has been paid to a correlation of the site of fluorescence with the histological characteristics of the fluorescing structures,[5,9-13] since this histological method offers an opportunity to investigate which cells possess and which cells are free from cytoplasmic or nuclear estrogen binding sites. Such a correlation was not found starting from the standard classification and biochemical values,[17] but a correlation could be established after technically complicated morphometric analysis of mammary tumor histology (see below).

Comparison of the results of various authors is difficult. They all describe the presence of cytoplasmic fluorescence, but seldom a detailed description of the fluorescing cells is given.

The presence of fluorescence of the nuclei is described by some authors as frequent, but others do not mention it at all. Seldom it is given more than a passing interest.

Concentrations in the incubation medium are difficult to compare, since the amount of bound estradiol and FITC varies. Usually the impression is gained that the medium is diluted until a satisfactory fluorescence is obtained. In many publications no mention is made of regular control of the presence of free estrogen or FITC in the incubation medium. Neither is an exact description of freezing and storing of the material found, nor the period between excision and freezing of the material, although it was demonstrated that these circumstances are paramount for the distribution and intensity of the fluorescence.[11,14]

Biochemically, three types of estrogen binding may be demonstrated in mammary tumors[18,19] which are designated type I, type II, and type III. These three estrogen binding entities become saturated with increasing estradiol concentrations in the incubation medium. Type I binding is saturated between $10^{-11}$ and $10^{-9}M$ estradiol, type II between $10^{-9}$ and $10^{-7}M$, and type III binding becomes saturated with concentrations above $10^{-7}M$. Accordingly, depending on the substrate concentration in the medium, type I binding dominates the amount of bound estradiol in concentrations below $10^{-9}M$ estradiol, type II binding between $10^{-9}$ and $10^{-7}M$, and above $10^{-7}M$ type III binding dominates the amount of estradiol bound. Biochemically, only the high-affinity binding saturable below $10^{-9}M$ is called the estrogen receptor proper. Lee,[1] in his first publication dealing with this subject, used the term estrogen receptor and implied that it was a type I receptor that was demonstrated. With regard to this assumption, or possibly without recognition of the problem, he was followed in various publications.[4,6,8,9,11] However, especially with regard to the identification of the fluorescence observed and the presence of type I receptors, other authors raised a number of pertinent questions.[7,12,16,18,20-25] According to the latter authors, the concentrations of the O-BSA-FITC complex in the incubation medium were too high to guarantee binding to type I receptors exclusively. Moreover, the number of type I receptors in one cell is too small to give a fluorescence observable with a standard epifluorescence system, even after a complete occupation of all receptors with a heavily FITC labeled O-BSA-FITC complex. Many O-BSA-FITC complexes appeared to be contaminated with free FITC and free estradiol, the latter sometimes in such high concentrations that all type I receptors would be occupied.[18,25] The concentrations of estradiol, diethylstilbestrol (DES) and antiestrogens, used to demonstrate the specificity of the reaction, also were too high for a specific competition with type I receptors only. All these critical observations, however, started from the same point, i.e., the only true receptor is the biochemically defined type I receptor and only binding to this receptor has clinical relevance.[7,18,20,23,25] No mention was made of the possibility that other binding sites (compare Reference 26) might have a scientific significance and clinical relevance of their own.

In this chapter discussed in some detail: (1) the specificity of the interaction between O-BSA-FITC* complex and thin sections of mammary tumors; (2) the correlation between morphological features of the mammary tumors and the presence of estrogen receptors assayed biochemically; and (3) the correlation between histochemical method and biochemical assay.

## II. SPECIFICITY OF THE INTERACTION BETWEEN O-BSA-FITC COMPLEX AND THIN SECTIONS OF MAMMARY TUMORS

Although it is known from the biochemical literature that the method of freezing, the temperature during, and the duration of storage affect the amount of demonstrable type I cytoplasmic estrogen receptors[27,28] in mammary tumors, in most publications concerning the interaction of an O-BSA-FITC complex and thin frozen sections no attention was paid to this phenomenon. Slow freezing and storage at temperatures above that of liquid nitrogen rapidly diminishes the amount of estrogen receptor binding sites.

It could be demonstrated that storage at room temperature or at 4°C for a period up to 1 hr has no or only a slight effect on the fluorescence observed. Storage at these temperatures during a longer period resulted in a very fast reduction of the number of fluorescing cells and intensity of the fluorescence as well as a deterioration of the histological picture.[70] The method of freezing determines the reproducibility of the fluorescence observed and its distribution.[14] Walker[11] also stresses that careful treatment of the tissue is essential to obtain reproducible results. If the material is frozen in large pieces or if it is frozen slowly, e.g., by placing it in an environment of −70°C or on a quick-freeze unit of a cryostat, a reduction or disappearance of binding of the O-BSA-FITC complex to a large part of the nuclei will be the result. Only rapid freezing with isopentane or freon cooled in liquid nitrogen maintains the binding capabilities. Both duration and temperature of the storage period are of consequence, too. Storage in liquid nitrogen (for periods over 1 year) has no influence on the distribution and intensity of the fluorescence. However, if properly frozen material is stored at higher temperatures (e.g., at −70°C) then both nuclear and cytoplasmic fluorescence disappear.[1,14] The fluorescence of the nuclei disappears first (already after 4 days, stored at −70°C), the fluorescence of the cytoplasm diminishes more slowly, but the majority of the fluorescence has disappeared as well after a fortnight storage at −70°C. Only the most

---

\* For convenience's sake only the designation O-BSA-FITC is used in this chapter, although markers other than FITC are used albeit less frequently. Walker[11] used horseradish peroxidase; Lee[10] used tetramethylrhodamine isothiocyanate in order to distinguish various steroid binding sites in one section simultaneously.

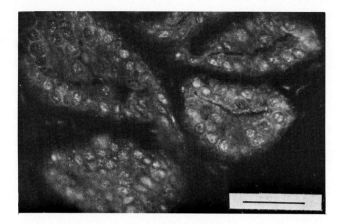

FIGURE 1.   In Figures 1 to 5, O-BSA-FITC induced fluorescence of premalignant mammary tissue and of mammary tumors. In order to facilitate comparison of the intensity of the fluorescence of the tumor cells, exposure and processing of all microphotographs took place under identical conditions. Scale: 50 μm.

intensively fluorescing cells (Figure 4) can still be observed. After sectioning of thin sections from the frozen tumor material they may be treated by freeze drying during 14 hr or a short dip in water-free acetone. Both methods provide a satisfactory conservation of the binding properties in nuclei as well as cytoplasm with respect to the O-BSA-FITC.

Differences among the various observations as to the presence or absence of fluorescence of the nuclei, variations in intensity of the fluorescence observed, and discrepancies in correlations of the fluorescence observed with the results of the biochemical estrogen receptor assay may be at least partly due to the facts described above and, hence, have their origin in differences of treatment of the material.

In order to demonstrate specific estrogen binding sites using an O-BSA-FITC complex in thin frozen sections of mammary tumors, first it should be confirmed that the interaction of estrogens with their specific binding sites is identical with the interaction of the O-BSA-FITC complex with these binding sites. It was established by Rao et al.[29] that the steroids covalently linked to BSA retain their ability to interact with their receptors and that the presence of FITC on the BSA did not interfere with the steroid-receptor interactions. Lee's suggestion that the number of steroid molecules bound to one molecule BSA is very critical[30] cannot be confirmed, from our own experiments[70] nor from the literature. Conjugates have been used with a varying number (4 to 28) of estradiol molecules bound to one molecule BSA and the reported results appear to be identical.[9,12,31]

Evaluation of the fluorescence present in thin sections from the frozen material of mammary tumors after incubation in an O-BSA-FITC-containing medium will give the following results, generally speaking. In most mammary tumors the density and intensity of fluorescence varies considerably, strongly fluorescing parts as well as less strongly fluorescing parts being found in the same tumor. Tumors showing no fluorescence at all are seldom encountered (about 2%).[1,3,5,6,9-11,13,14] Sections from the periphery of the tumor display more positive cells and a more pronounced fluorescence than sections from the more central parts. Not only mammary tumors but premalignant mammary tissue as well will show a fluorescence after incubation. Positive cytoplasm and nuclei are both (Figure 1) encountered, but their fluorescence is not as pronounced as in most tumors.

The fluorescence may be present in the nucleus as well as in the cytoplasm of the tumor cells (Figures 2 to 5). If present, the fluorescence of the nucleus is very often much more

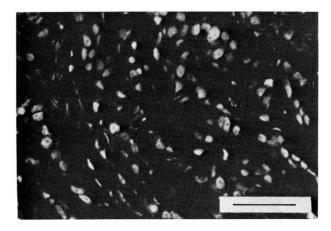

FIGURE 2.   Infiltrating tumor with fluorescence predominantly located in the nuclei.

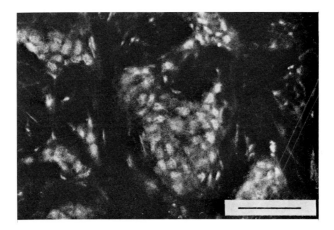

FIGURE 3.   Infiltrating tumor with fluorescence in the nuclei as well as in the cytoplasm.

intense than the fluorescence of the cytoplasm (Figures 2 and 3).[4,9,11,14] Especially intra-ductally growing tumors with large cells show a pronounced cytoplasmic fluorescence, whereas the nuclear fluorescence is absent (Figure 4). Particularly in this type of tumors occasionally single scattered cells are observed with a much more pronounced fluorescence than their surrounding cells. Other intraductally growing tumors with only slightly smaller cells show a well-developed fluorescence of the cytoplasm and the nuclei (Figure 5).

Mammary tumors with small cells often show a pronounced nuclear fluorescence which is sometimes so intense that it is difficult to observe and to estimate the intensity of cyto-plasmic fluorescence (Figure 2). Especially the fluorescence of this type of tumors is affected by inadequate freezing.[14] Contrary to the large cell tumors which show scattered cells that are far more fluorescent than their neighbors, these infiltrating tumors are remarkably ho-mogeneous regarding the intensity of the fluorescence of the nucleus as well as the cytoplasm. Cells with a markedly different nuclear or cytoplasmic fluorescence are hardly observed.

The fact that various authors confirmed the aforementioned observations and reported the reproducibility of the results is an indication that, indeed, a specific interaction takes place between the O-BSA-FITC complex and the frozen sections of the mammary tumors.[3]

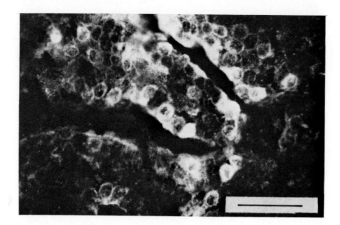

FIGURE 4.   Intraductal tumor with fluorescence located exclusively in the cytoplasm.

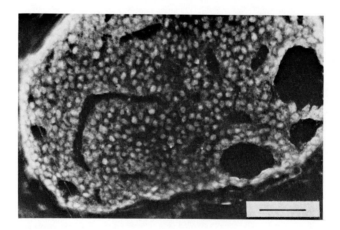

FIGURE 5.   Intraductal tumor with fluorescence located in the nuclei and in the cytoplasm.

The arguments presented below may also support the hypothesis that the interaction between the O-BSA-FITC complex and the sections is specific and determined by the presence of estrogen binding sites in the section.

The use of incubation media with varying concentrations of the O-BSA-FITC complex (between $10^{-7}$ and $5 \times 10^{-9}$ $M$) does not change the distribution of the fluorescence.[14] Only the intensity of the fluorescence diminishes at decreasing concentrations, however, a change in the relative intensities is not observed. Since prolonged washing of the sections after incubation has no effect on the intensity or the localization of the fluorescence,[14,26] we may assume that only very little aspecific binding is present[14,26] and that it is not the aspecific binding which is the origin of the fluorescence observed.[21] In our hands an incubation medium containing $5 \times 10^{-9}M$ O-BSA-FITC appeared to be the lowest concentration for obtaining a fluorescence in the sections just observable using a normal fluorescence system with epi-illumination.[14] Incubation media containing more than $10^{-7}$ $M$ complex produce an aspecific staining of various structures according to our experience. Prolonged washing (12 hr) after incubation in a medium with such a high concentration of the complex causes a conspicuous reduction of the fluorescence of most structures; some structures even become negative (e.g., connective tissue, blood vessels).

From these findings the conclusion may be drawn that when concentrations of the O-BSA-FITC complex between $5 \times 10^{-9}$ and $10^{-7}$ are used, a high affinity appears to exist between the complex and the binding sites in thin sections of the mammary tumors.

That the binding of the O-BSA-FITC complex is specific for estradiol could be demonstrated. Binding of the complex to thin sections is inhibited by various antiestrogens,[4,6,9,11,14] free diethylstilbestrol (DES),[4,9,11,13,26] and free estradiol.[1,4,10,14,26] An explanation for the partial inhibition mentioned by some authors[1,4,13,14] was offered by Lee.[26] He demonstrated that a complete inhibition could be obtained using prolonged incubation periods[26] and that the partial inhibition was due to the incubation periods being too short.

The estrogen binding sites in the sections are the only sites involved in the binding of the O-BSA-FITC complex to the sections. This can be demonstrated by the addition of progesterone, androsterone, or testosterone to the incubation medium. Their presence in a 100 or 200 $\times$ mol excess concentration does not influence the fluorescence of the sections in any respect.[4,9,10,70]

From the facts presented above we may conclude that from a histochemical point of view the interaction of the O-BSA-FITC complex with the thin frozen sections demonstrates the presence of binding sites specific for estradiol combined with a high affinity for estradiol[3] and not an aspecific interaction with tissue proteins.[21] The term estrogen binding sites was used by Hanna et al.[13] Most publications report a good correlation between the presence of these binding sites (usually called receptors) in mammary tumors and the biochemical cytosol values,[4,6,8,9,11,13,15] although some report that such a correlation is absent.[5,7,12] The biochemical identity of these binding sites is a point in question. As stated already above three types of estrogen binding can be demonstrated, i.e., type I, type II, and III,[18] and only type I binding which is saturable between $10^{-11}$ and $10^{-9}$ $M$ is called the receptor proper. In accordance with increasing estrogen concentrations, type I (between $10^{-11}$ and $10^{-9}$ $M$), type II ($10^{-9}$ to $10^{-7}$ $M$), and type III (above $10^{-7}$ $M$), respectively, dominate the amount of bound estrogen. Considering the concentration of the O-BSA-FITC complex in the incubation medium (nearly always above $10^{-8}$ $M$), the assumption is justified that apart from type I binding type II and III binding are involved as well.[18,25] At the same time the argument is valid that too little type I receptors are present in the cytoplasm to present sufficient fluorescence to be detectable with a normal epifluorescence system, even if completely occupied with a heavily FITC labeled complex.[18] Other arguments concerning the aspecificity of the interaction are (1) the solubility of the type I receptors; (2) in many instances the inhibition reported is only partial; (3) high concentrations of DES, antiestrogens, and estradiol are necessary to obtain an inhibition.*

Lee[26] investigated the binding of O-BSA-FITC to thin frozen sections of mammary tumors. He was able to demonstrate that in the sections type I binding was still present, and his conclusion is that the cytosol assay demonstrates only the soluble part of type I receptors in the cytoplasm. The majority of the type I receptor is membrane bound and is not demonstrated with the biochemical assay. He was able, also, to demonstrate that partial inhibition with DES as reported in the literature[1,4,9,12] was due to the incubation periods being too short. Incubation periods of 16 hr or longer produced a complete inhibition of the binding. If antiestrogens are used to inhibit the interaction of O-BSA-FITC with the section, longer incubation times will probably also produce a complete inhibition. Consequently, part of

---

\* In this discussion we do not comment on impurities (unbound estradiol and FITC) of the O-BSA-FITC complex as discussed extensively elsewhere.[18] since these problems can be solved keeping a rigorous control on the synthesis. From the limited experience the authors had with various commercial samples they could not but conclude that all samples were contaminated with free estradiol and FITC.

the criticism would be the result of the application of biochemical criteria, valid for reactions taking place in solution, to the completely different conditions of binding to a solid substrate (the frozen section).[26] These different conditions would be an explanation for long incubation times and high concentrations necessary to obtain a complete inhibition. They may also explain the reported differences in affinity of the O-BSA-FITC complex to estrogen binding sites. Lee[26] reports an affinity of the complex to binding sites comparable to DES, whereas McCarty et al.[7] and Joyce et al.[12] report a binding affinity about $10^{-4} \times$ the affinity of DES for type I binding in a cytosol preparation. Considering the high affinity of the O-BSA-FITC complex for the binding sites, prolonged washing has no effect on the fluorescence and the specificity of the binding. Lee[26] concludes that only type I binding might explain the binding of the O-BSA-FITC complex to sections.

Binding of the O-BSA-FITC complex to type II binding sites is considered improbable by Lee,[26] since type II binding would not be resistant to prolonged washings.[32]

In view of the explanation presented above it should be stressed, and Lee rightly observed,[26] that the type I binding described is totally different (i.e., membrane bound) from the soluble type I receptors demonstrated with the biochemical cytosol assay. This also implies that, according to Lee's conclusion, using the cytosol assay only a small part, i.e., only the soluble fraction of the type I receptors, is demonstrated.

Although this is not favored by Lee,[26] other authors[12,14] try to explain the binding of O-BSA-FITC complex to the presence of type II binding sites in the thin frozen sections of mammary tumors.

Clark et al.[33,34] demonstrated a cytoplasmic estradiol binding in the cytosol of the rat uterus saturable between $10^{-9}$ and $10^{-7}$ $M$. Similar to type I binding the binding of estradiol to type II receptors could be inhibited by DES. That this binding is inhibited by antiestrogens is probable and this interaction is possibly described by Clark et al. and Murphy et al.[35,36] in rat uteri. A reduction of the binding resulting in a reduction or complete disappearance of the fluorescence owing to antiestrogens or DES, consequently, does not prove that only type I binding (i.e., the estradiol receptor proper) is involved in the interaction of the O-BSA-FITC complex with the sections. A direct indication of the involvement of type II binding is the observation that in the presence of dithiothreitol a marked reduction of the fluorescence took place.[12] Accordingly, binding of the O-BSA-FITC complex to thin sections of the rat uterus may be explained by the interaction of type II binding sites with the complex. Panko et al.[19] demonstrated the presence of type II binding in mammary tumors in large amounts. Considering the concentrations of O-BSA-FITC in the medium and the effect of thiothreitol, the presumptive explanation of the interaction of sections of mammary tumors with the complex is that it is at least partly due to an interaction with type II binding sites. If this explanation would be accepted, it could also serve as an explanation for the close correlation between histochemical and biochemical results.

Panko et al.[19] demonstrated a positive relationship between the amount of type I and type II binding. The more type I binding present in the cytosol, the more type II binding was found. Demonstration and estimation of type II binding is also an indication of the amount of type I binding, i.e., of the estrogen receptor.

Although various authors described the presence of fluorescing nuclei, little attention has been paid to this phenomenon. Neither the significance nor the specificity of the reaction are discussed in detail. As with the cytoplasmic fluorescence it may be argued that from a histological point of view a specific binding is obtained, since the fluorescence is resistant to prolonged washing (unpublished observations), can be reduced or abolished with antiestrogens, and is not affected by the presence of testosterone, progesterone, and androsterone. The observation that after administration of estradiol or the antiestrogen tamoxifen in vivo the fluorescence of the nuclei of rat uteri is increased,[12] supports the conclusion of a specific binding insofar that it is a physiological phenomenon that is observed, since tamoxifen is known to increase the nuclear amount of type II estrogen binding sites.[37]

In view of the high concentration of the O-BSA-FITC complex we are inclined to ascribe the fluorescence observed in the nuclei to binding of the O-BSA-FITC complex to type II estrogen binding sites, although we must admit that further investigation will be necessary to elucidate the exact nature of the binding of the O-BSA-FITC complex to nuclei in thin frozen sections.

It has been reported[12,38] that after incubation of sections of mammary tumors in BSA-FITC, a fluorescence is observed indistinguishable from the fluorescence which develops after incubation in O-BSA-FITC. In other words, a large amount of the fluorescence observed after incubation in O-BSA-FITC would be aspecific. However, further investigation of this phenomenon provided the following data. Not all batches of commercially obtained BSA show the above-mentioned properties to an equal degree after coupling to FITC. Some batches show a marked fluorescence, others are negative or slightly positive. The fluorescence developed is resistant to prolonged washing, shows a distribution completely identical with the O-BSA-FITC fluorescence, whereas other steroids than estrogens do not affect the fluorescence, while the BSA-FITC fluorescence is abolished in the presence of antiestrogens or high concentrations of estradiol.[14,70] Considering these properties the only conclusion we can draw is that the observations mentioned are not due to faulty chemical procedures as was suggested,[39] but to estradiol bound to some batches of serum albumin. Estrogens are known to bind to albumins[40] and commercially obtained samples may be contaminated in various degrees.

From the results published in the literature so far it cannot be established without doubt which type of biochemically defined estrogen binding is demonstrated with the histochemical O-BSA-FITC method. Type I as well as type II binding must be taken into consideration. However, if, indeed, type I binding is demonstrated as is suggested,[26] then it is different from the type I binding biochemically assayed.

Whatever estrogen binding is demonstrated histochemically the binding sites demonstrated are membrane bound. Considering the good reproducibility of the histochemical method and the specificity and high affinity of the estrogen binding site demonstrated, the O-BSA-FITC method has its own value as a research tool. However, its use as an indication to hormonal therapy as is established for the biochemical assay awaits further investigation.

## III. CORRELATION BETWEEN MORPHOLOGICAL FEATURES OF THE MAMMARY TUMORS AND THE PRESENCE OF ESTROGEN RECEPTORS ASSAYED BIOCHEMICALLY

In several studies a significant correlation has been found between the presence of estrogen receptors and histological parameters of primary breast cancer. Histological features such as histologic type, histologic grade, nuclear grade, and degree of elastosis[41,42] can be assessed with a subjectively microscopic evaluation. Usually these qualitatively subjective features are graded in three categories, viz., histologic grade I, II, and III. If for 198 patients the presence or absence of estrogen receptors is plotted against the histologic grade, a correlation (or confusion) matrix is obtained which may appear as follows:

| | Histologic grade | | | |
| --- | --- | --- | --- | --- |
| | III | II | I | Total |
| Estrogen receptor negative | 21 | 17 | 6 | 44 |
| Estrogen receptor positive | 30 | 93 | 31 | 154 |
| Total | 51 | 110 | 37 | 198 |

From this matrix the conclusion can be drawn that histologic grade I tumors (well-differentiated cancers) are much more often estrogen receptor positive than badly or nondifferentiated grade III tumors. This difference is statistically highly significant (pChi 2 = 0.0008). However, the matrix also shows a considerable overlap, e.g., many grade I tumors are estrogen receptor negative and a number of grade III tumors are estrogen receptor positive. The same phenomenon is found in other qualitatively subjective features. Hence, the predictive value of these features is not very high and their practical usefulness is limited.

Part of this overlap may be the result of inconsistencies owing to the subjective assessment of the grading, and in principle this difficulty can be overcome by quantitative microscopy. This has the advantage of objectivity, reproducibility, and consistency.

It has been demonstrated that, generally speaking, estrogen receptor positive tumors contain smaller nuclei and are more cellular than estrogen receptor negative ones, independent of histological type.[43,44] Parallel findings are found in cytological specimens. Recently these findings could be confirmed.[45] The additional value of morphometry in assessing qualitative features as histologic, nuclear, and elastosis grades has been investigated, using single- and multivariate analysis. These statistical techniques may add considerably to the discriminating power of morphometry.[46] An outline is given below of the best combination of qualitative and/or morphometric predictors of estrogen receptors in breast cancer.

## A. Methodology

The charcoal method was applied for the detection of estrogen receptor activity.[47]

For qualitative and quantitative microscopy, 4-$\mu$m paraffin sections stained with hematoxylin eosin or with the Verhoef modification of the elastine stain were used. Histologic grades were evaluated as indicated by Bloom[48] and subsequent authors,[49,50] while for nuclear grading the criteria of Black and Speer[51] were applied. Elastosis was graded as 0 if the stroma between the neoplastic cells was completely negative; as II if the stroma around the neoplastic cells was markedly positive, and as grade I if there was an intermediate degree of elastine fiber formation. This elastosis grading provided the following results: 20% of all 198 cases appeared to be negative, 40% showed grade I, and 40% grade II.

Mitotic activity, cellularity index, and qualitative nuclear parameters as mean nuclear area, standard deviation of the nuclear area, were assessed quantitatively as described by Baak et al.[45,52]

## B. Results

There is a definite dependence between age and estrogen receptor content in the 198 cases studied. With an approximate distinction line at age 50 years, patients on or below this line have a smaller estrogen receptor content than patients above this line. Since multivariate analysis can be applied only to approximately homogeneous groups, the two age groups were investigated separately with age 50 as distinction line. The group below or equal to 50 years numbered 60, the group above 50 years numbered 138.[45]

In general, it appeared that estrogen receptor positive tumors demonstrate a lower histologic grade (i.e., more normal appearing glands), a higher nuclear grade (i.e., less pleomorphic nuclei), and a higher elastosis grade. Moreover, they are more cellular and contain smaller nuclei. Elastosis appeared to be the best single discriminator in patients above 50 years, whereas in patients equal to or below 50 years the morphometrically assessed features are better discriminators, especially the mean and standard deviation of the nuclear area. In Figure 6 the mean and standard deviation of the nuclear area for patients equal to or below 50 years are plotted on the X and Y axis, respectively. If the dotted lines are used as decision threshold, so that the cases in the lower left corner of the figure will be regarded positive, in the upper right corner negative, and between the decision lines as doubtful, a satisfactory prediction is obtained in patients below 51 years. This prediction using morphometric features

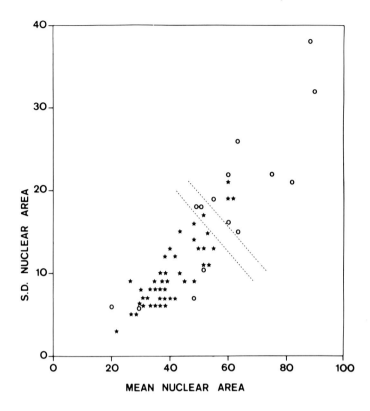

FIGURE 6. Distinction between estrogen receptor positive tumors (asterisks) and negative tumors (circles) in patients age below 51 years related to two morphometrical features, i.e., standard deviation (SD) of the nuclear area and mean nuclear area ($\mu m^2$). (Reproduced from Baak, J. P. A. and Persijn, J., *Pathol. Res. Pract.*, in press. With permission.)

is more reliable than predictors on qualitatively subjective features as histologic, nuclear, and elastosis grade. In patients over 50 years of age a multivariate analysis of both the morphometric and the qualitatively subjective features showed that a combination of degree of elastosis and mean nuclear area, according to the decision tree in Figure 7, is the optimal predictor combination for the presence of estrogen receptors. (A more detailed treatise on this subject has already been published.[45])

Although not a predictor of primary importance, the measured mitotic activity was significantly higher in estrogen receptor negative tumors than in estrogen receptor positive tumors. This agrees with the results of Olszewski et al.[55,56] and the data of Meijer et al.[57] The first described that mammary tumors with low DNA ploidy tended to be estrogen receptor positive, while those with high DNA ploidy tended to be negative; the second demonstrated using thymidine incorporation that breast cancers with a high rate of proliferation have few estrogen receptors.

## C. Comments

The reliability of the developed morphometric classification indicates the possibility to use these methods as a (second choice) technique to predict the presence or absence of estrogen receptors in mammary tumors in cases where it is not possible to use the biochemical charcoal assay. Although in patients equal to or below 50 years an outspoken correlation exists between the mean and the standard deviation of the nuclear area of mammary tumors and the presence of estrogen receptors, such a correlation is lacking in patients older than

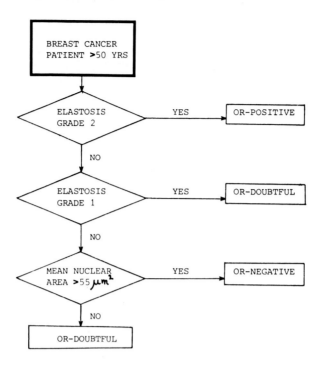

FIGURE 7.   Decision tree for the evaluation of estrogen receptors in patients age over 50. (Reproduced from Baak, J. P. A. and Persijn, J., *Pathol. Res. Pract.*, 1984. With permission.)

50 years. For this discrepancy we cannot forward a definite explanation. Considering the differences between the below/equal 50-years group and the above 50-years group it is surprising that these differences were not noted before and that in previous studies all patients were treated as one group irrespective of age.

## IV. CORRELATION BETWEEN HISTOCHEMICAL METHOD AND BIOCHEMICAL ASSAY

There is a general agreement on the assumption that there is a positive correlation between the presence of estrogen receptors in breast cancer and a prolonged disease-free interval.[58,59] Moreover, estrogen receptor-rich breast cancers appear more likely to respond to endocrine therapy than to chemotherapy.[59,60] Usually estrogen receptors are determined using biochemical assays of which the competitive protein binding assay (dextran-coated charcoal method)[47,61] is the most important.

The biochemical assay has the advantage of a numerical value, but it requires homogenization of the generally heterogeneous tissue specimens. Problems of variability and reproducibility are prone to occur, while the method itself is relatively expensive and laborious. Varying localization of the estrogen receptors in tumor cells, sampling errors, and necrotic areas may cause erroneous results. These disadvantages of the biochemical methods have led to a cytochemical approach in order to demonstrate estrogen receptors in frozen tissue sections.[10,18,62]

Histochemical assays are relatively easy to perform. However, demonstration of a correlation between biochemical assays and histochemical assays have been hampered by difficulties in interpretation of the results of the histochemical assay. Moreover, the specificity of the histochemical assays has been questioned. Problems of interpretation as regards the histochemical assays are

1.   The percentage of estrogen receptor positive tumor cells in breast carcinoma may vary considerably.
2.   The estrogen receptor content in nuclei and/or cytoplasm in tumor cell often differs from one cell to another.

Of great potential value is the recently developed isoelectric focusing assay for estrogen receptors in cryostat sections.[69] It allows a very close comparison of quantitative histology of mammary tumors, estrogen receptor content, and histochemical demonstration of estrogen binding sites, and it minimizes sampling errors, etc.

Correlating of the biochemical assay and the histochemical method poses an extra problem, viz., the variation of the percentages of tumor cells in a tissue block of tumor. Thus, prerequisites for a study comparing biochemical assays and histochemical methods are

1.   Demonstration of the specificity of the histochemical assay.
2.   Definition of criteria for the interpretation of histochemical results.
3.   Histological control of the tissue specimens used for the biochemical assay to exclude sampling errors and necrotic areas.

In the various publications dealing with a correlation of biochemical assay and histochemical assay,[6,7,9,15,26,62,63] a positive correlation was found only in some.[6,15,62,63] However, although these groups are aware of the problems complicating the interpretation of the histochemical results, criteria for the interpretation of these histochemical results are not clearly defined in all publications. Recently we described in detail a histochemical assay for the demonstration and quantification of estrogen receptors in frozen sections using 17β-estradiol-6-carboxymethyloxime bovine serum albumin-FITC (O-BSA-FITC).[14,15]

This method using three dilutions (1:20, 1:40, 1:80) of the O-BSA-FITC complex (concentration $5 \times 10^{-6} M$) demonstrates at least type II receptors[14] and allows a semiquantitative estimation of the intensity of fluorescence (Table 1).

Since a positive correlation is demonstrated between type I and type II receptors in mammary tumors[19] as discussed above, a quantification of both the number of fluorescing cells and the intensity of the fluorescence is also an estimate of the amount of type I estrogen receptors present in the tissue specimen. Using strictly defined criteria for interpretation of the histochemical results, we have compared in 132 breast carcinomas and 12 benign breast specimens with varying degree of mastopathic changes the results of such a histochemical assay with those of the charcoal method.

## A. Technical Details

Values obtained by the charcoal method larger than 11,000 fmol/g protein were classified as estrogen receptor positive and values smaller than 9,000 fmol/g protein were classified as estrogen receptor negative. Values between 9,000 and 11,000 fmol/g protein were considered doubtful.

In each histochemical assay human uterus and benign breast specimens were used as positive controls. After reading the fluorescence of the sections in a number of cases sections were fixed in Carnoy's fixative and stained with hematoxylin eosin to evaluate the histological structures. After incubation in diluted O-BSA-FITC medium three parameters were determined:

1.   The percentage of epithelial structures with respect to the total amount of tissue; this was done semiquantitatively.[64]
2.   The percentage of fluorescing epithelial cells; a cell was considered to have a positive fluorescence with a nucleus and/or cytoplasm showing fluorescence.

**Table 1**
## SEMIQUANTITATIVE ESTIMATION OF THE INTENSITY OF FLUORESCENCE

| Dilution[a] O-BSA-FITC | (conc 5 × 10⁻⁶) | Intensity of fluorescence | | | | |
|---|---|---|---|---|---|---|
| 1:20 | | + + | + + | + / + + | + | + / − |
| 1:40 | | + + | + | + | + / − | − |
| 1:80 | | + | + | − | − | − |
| Degree of intensity of fluorescence indicated as | | IV | III | II | I | 0 |

*Note:*  − = negative, + = positive, and + + = strongly positive.

[a]   O-BSA-FITC = 17β-estradiol-6 carboxymethyloxime bovine serum albumen-FITC.

3.   The degree of intensity of fluorescence was graded semiquantitatively from I to IV as follows: in three dilutions (1:20, 1:40, and 1:80) of the O-BSA-FITC complex (concentration 5 × 10⁻⁶ $M$) the intensity of fluorescence was estimated varying from negative ( − ) to positive ( + ) to strongly positive ( + + ).

Table 1 shows how the fluorescence was graded. When groups of cells were present with different intensities of fluorescence, the total percentage of fluorescing cells was recorded with the lowest intensity found. This was done because the percentages of fluorescing tumor cells with stronger intensity of fluorescence varied in the majority of cases between 0 and 10%.

## B. Criteria for the Interpretation of Results of Histochemical Assay

Histochemically, a tumor was considered estrogen receptor negative when (1) degree I or less intensity of fluorescence was found irrespective of the percentage of fluorescing tumor cells; or (2) when 10% or less of the tumor cells showed fluorescence irrespective of the intensity of fluorescence. A tumor was marked estrogen receptor doubtful when 20 or 30% of the tumor cells showed degree II of intensity of fluorescence.

Estrogen receptor was marked positive: (1) when 20% or more of the tumor cells with intensity of fluorescence degree III or more were observed; or (2) when 40% or more of the tumor cells with intensity of fluorescence degree II or more were observed.

Reading of the estrogen receptor-stained slides was done independently by two pathologists. These two readings showed no discrepancies.

## C. Results and Concluding Remarks

Before homogenization of the tissue specimens for biochemical assay three cryostat sections (4 μm) were made of the tissue to be used for biochemical assay in order to determine whether and how many tumor cells were present in the tissue specimens. Table 2 and Figure 8 show a good correlation between the histochemical assay and the charcoal method. Moreover, Figure 8 presents a semiquantitative impression of the intensity of fluorescence. In general, there was a tendency for high estrogen receptor values in the biochemical assay to correlate with higher numbers of tumor cells showing a high degree (III and IV) intensity of fluorescence.

Table 3 lists the specimens which led to disagreement between charcoal method and histochemical assay. From the results with benign and malignant breast specimens it was interpreted that when the percentage of the epithelial structures in a specimen was lower than 15% the estrogen receptor content in the biochemical assay was always negative. The

**Table 2**
## CORRELATION BETWEEN THE CHARCOAL METHOD AND HISTOCHEMICAL ASSAY (n = 132)

| | | Negative | Doubtful | Positive |
|---|---|---|---|---|
| Charcoal method | Negative | 30 | 0 | 5 |
| | Doubtful | 0 | 2 | 2 |
| | Positive | 3 | 1 | 89 |

| | | |
|---|---|---|
| Agreement | 121 cases = | 91.6% |
| Slight disagreement | 3 cases = | 2.3% |
| Disagreement | 8 cases = | 6.1% |

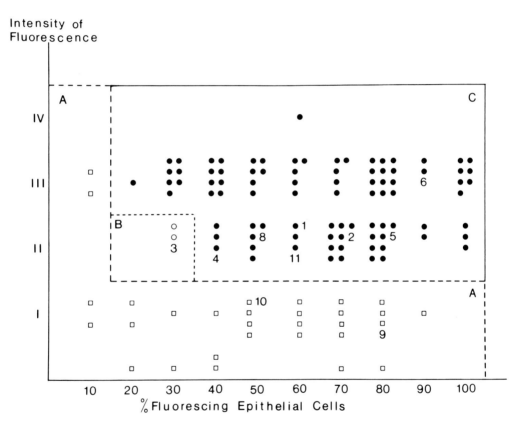

FIGURE 8. Correlation between histochemically and biochemically determined estrogen receptors (n = 131). One case is not recorded because no epithelial structures were found in the tissue specimen used for the histochemical assay (see case no. 7, Table 5). The numbers in the figure represent the cases in which differences were found between the results of the histochemical and those of the biochemical assay. These numbers correspond with the numbers of the cases in Table 5. Compartment A = histochemically negative (— — —); compartment B = histochemically doubtful (- - - -); compartment C = histochemically positive (————); ● = biochemically positive; ○ = biochemically doubtful; □ = biochemically negative.

reason may be the impossibility to express an estrogen receptor content in the biochemical assay in femtomole per gram protein epithelial structure instead of femtomole per gram protein tissue. It appeared that in the majority of cases these discrepancies between the results of the charcoal method and the histochemical assay were caused by sampling errors of the tissue specimens and a low volume percentage of epithelial structures in the tissue

## Table 3
### ESTROGEN RECEPTOR ACTIVITY IN 11 INFILTRATING DUCT CARCINOMAS WITH DISAGREEMENT BETWEEN THE CHARCOAL METHOD AND HISTOCHEMICAL ASSAY

| Specimen no. | Age (years) | Protein (fmol/g) | Conclusion (charcoal method) | Fluorescing epithelial cells (%) | Intensity of fluorescence | Volume percent of epithelium | Conclusion (histochemical method) | Remarks |
|---|---|---|---|---|---|---|---|---|
| 1 | 58 | 9,600 | Doubtful | 60 | II | <15 | Positive | A, lymph node metastasis |
| 2 | 63 | 3,200 | Negative | 70 | II | <15 | Positive | A |
| 3 | 72 | 18,000 | Postive | 30 | II | 40 | Doubtful | No explanation |
| 4 | 61 | 6,900 | Negative | 40 | II | <15 | Positive | A |
| 5 | 57 | 4,300 | Negative | 80 | II | 40 | Positive | B |
| 6 | 38 | 3,900 | Negative | 90 | III | 30 | Positive | B |
| 7 | 78 | 230,000 | Positive | — | — | — | Negative | Tissue specimen for histochemical assay contained no epithelial cells |
| 8 | 41 | 9,300 | Doubtful | 50 | II | 20 | Positive | No explanation |
| 9 | 59 | 12,000 | Positive | 80 | I | 50 | Negative | Lymph node metastasis |
| 10 | 37 | 13,000 | Positive | 50 | I | 60 | Negative | Myoepithelium estrogen receptor positive |
| 11 | 86 | 6,000 | Negative | 60 | II | 50 | Positive | B |

*Note:*   A = percentage of epithelial structures in tissue specimen used for histochemical and biochemical assay too low ($<15\%$) to find biochemically estrogen receptor activity; B = percentage of epithelial structures in tissue specimen used for biochemical assay lower than 15%.

specimens, as has also been demonstrated by Pertschuk et al. and Walker et al.[6,62] The presence of estrogen receptor positive myoepithelial cells proved to be another factor causing discrepancy. Presence of necrosis, however, as is mentioned[1,62,63] was not considered an important disturbing factor, probably because in our setting the pathologists instead of clinicians select the tissue specimens which were sent to the biochemical laboratory.

Two other notes are important in this context. It is known from the literature that only 60 to 70% of the patients with biochemically determined positive estrogen receptor respond to endocrine therapy.[65] Preliminary observations[6,62] indicate that certain groups of breast carcinomas with only nuclear estrogen receptors have a bad prognosis. Hence, it may well be that the use of the histochemical assay for the detection of estrogen receptor activity may improve our ability to predict the response to endocrine therapy, not only by demonstrating the absence of estrogen receptor activity, but also by detecting certain groups of tumor cells with characteristic patterns of estrogen receptor.

In addition, many workers feel that the quantity of estrogen receptor is related to prognosis, i.e., the greater the receptor concentration as demonstrated biochemically, the better the response to therapy and the better the prognosis.[66-68]

Never in the literature has a direct correlation been brought forward between the histochemical results and clinical data. Hence, studies in which a direct correlation between the histochemical results and clinical response to therapy and prognosis is evaluated are important because the histochemical method has a high potential value in its use for small-needle biopsies and cytologic material.

# REFERENCES

1. **Lee, S. H.,** Cytochemical study of estrogen receptor in human mammary cancer, *Am. J. Clin. Pathol.,* 70, 197, 1978.
2. **Buell, R. H. and Tremblay, G.,** Autoradiographic demonstration of uptake and retention of ³H-estradiol after in vitro incubation, *J. Histochem. Cytochem.,* 29, 1316, 1981.
3. **Nenci, I.,** Estrogen receptor cytochemistry in human breast cancer. Status and prospects, *Cancer,* 48, 2674, 1981.
4. **Pertschuk, L. P., Gaetjens, E., Carter, A. C., Brigati, D. J., Kim, D. S., and Fealey, T. E.,** An improved histochemical method for detection of estrogen receptors in mammary cancer. Comparison with biochemical assay, *Am. J. Clin. Pathol.,* 71, 504, 1979.
5. **Lee, S. H.,** Cancer cell estrogen receptor of human mammary carcinoma, *Cancer,* 44, 1, 1979.
6. **Walker, R. A., Cove, D. H., and Howell, A.,** Histological detection of oestrogen receptor in human breast carcinomas, *Lancet,* 1, 171, 1980.
7. **McCarty, K. S., Woodard, B. H., Nichols, D. E., Wilkinson, W., and McCarty, K. S.,** Comparison of biochemical and histochemical techniques for estrogen receptor analyses in mammary carcinoma, *Cancer,* 46, 2842, 1980.
8. **Pertschuk, L. P., Tobin, E. H., Gaetjens, E., Carter, A. C., Degenshein, G. A., Bloom, N. D., and Brigati, D. J.,** Histochemical assay of estrogen and progesterone receptors in breast cancer, *Cancer,* 46, 2896, 1980.
9. **Pertschuk, L. P., Tobin, E. H., Tanapat, P., Gaetjens, E., Carter, A. C., Bloom, N. D., Macchia, R. J., and Eisenberg, K. B.,** Histochemical analyses of steroid hormone receptors in breast and prostatic carcinoma, *J. Histochem. Cytochem.,* 28, 799, 1980.
10. **Lee, S. H.,** Cellular estrogen and progesterone receptors in mammary carcinoma, *Am. J. Clin. Pathol.,* 73, 323, 1980.
11. **Walker, R. A.,** The cytochemical demonstration of oestrogen receptors in human breast carcinomas, *J. Pathol.,* 135, 237, 1981.
12. **Joyce, B. G., Nicholson, R. I., Morton, M. S., and Griffiths, K.,** Studies with steroid-fluorescein conjugates on oestrogen target tissues, *Eur. J. Cancer Clin. Oncol.,* 18, 1147, 1982.
13. **Hanna, W., Ryder, D. E., and Mobbs, B. G.,** Cellular localization of estrogen binding sites in human breast cancer, *Am. J. Clin. Pathol.,* 77, 391, 1982.

14. **van Marle, J., Lindeman, J., Ariëns, A. Th., Labruyère, W., and Van Weeren-Kramer, J.,** Estrogen receptors in human breast cancer. I. Specificity of the histochemical localization of estrogen receptors using an estrogen-albumin FITC complex, *Virchows Arch. (Cell Pathol.),* 40, 17, 1982.

15. **Meijer, C. J. L. M., van Marle, J., Persijn, J. P., Van Nieuwenhuizen, W., Baak, J.P. A., Boon, M. E., and Lindeman, J.,** Estrogen receptors in human breast cancer. II. Correlation between histochemical method and biochemical assay, *Virchows Arch. (Cell Pathol.),* 40, 27, 1982.

16. **Panko, W. B., Mattioli, C. A., and Wheeler, T. M.,** Lack of correlation of a histochemical method for estrogen receptor analysis with the biochemical assay results, *Cancer,* 49, 2148, 1982.

17. **DeSombre, E. R., Carbone, P. P., Jensen, E. V., McGuire, W. L., Wells, S. A., Wittliff, J. L., and Lipsett, M. B.,** Steroid receptors in breast cancer, *N. Engl. J. Med.,* 301, 1011, 1979.

18. **Chamness, G. C., Mercer, W. D., and McGuire, W. L.,** Are histochemical methods for estrogen receptor valid, *J. Histochem. Cytochem.,* 28, 792, 1980.

19. **Panko, W. B., Watson, C. S., and Clark, J. H.,** The presence of a second, specific estrogen binding site in human breast cancer, *J. Steroid Biochem.,* 14, 1311, 1981.

20. **Penney, G. C. and Hawkins, R. A.,** Histochemical assay of oestrogen receptor, *Lancet,* 1, 930, 1980.

21. **Katzenellenbogen, J. A., Heiman, D. F., Carlson, K. E., Payne, D. W., and Lloyd, J. E.,** Optimization of the binding selectivity of estrogens, in *Cytotoxic Estrogens in Hormone Receptive Tumors,* Raus, J., Martens, H., and Leclercq, G., Eds., Academic Press, New York, 1980, 3.

22. **Stumpf, W. E. and Sar, M.,** Histochemical approaches for the localization of steroid hormone receptors, *Acta Histochem. Cytochem.,* 15, 560, 1982.

23. **Chamness, G. C. and McGuire, W. L.,** Questions about histochemical methods for steroid receptors, *Arch. Pathol. Lab. Med.,* 106, 53, 1982.

24. **Stumpf, W. E.,** The histochemistry of steroid hormone "receptors", *J. Histochem. Cytochem.,* 31, 113, 1983.

25. **Underwood, J. C. E., Sher, E., Reed, M., Eisman, J. A., and Martin, T. J.,** Biochemical assessment of histochemical methods for oestrogen receptor localisation, *J. Clin. Pathol.,* 35, 401, 1982.

26. **Lee, S. H.,** The histochemistry of estrogen receptors, *Histochemistry,* 71, 491, 1981.

27. **Namkung, P. C., Moe, R. E., and Petra, P. H.,** Stability of estrogen receptors in frozen human breast tumor tissue, *Cancer Res.,* 39, 1124, 1979.

28. **Muschenheim, F., Furst, J. L., and Bates, H. A.,** Increased incidence of positive tests for estrogen binding in mammary carcinoma specimens transported in liquid nitrogen, *Am. J. Clin. Pathol.,* 70, 780, 1978.

29. **Rao, B. R., Patrick, T. B., and Sweet, F.,** Steroid-albumin conjugate interaction with steroid-binding proteins, *Endocrinology,* 106, 356, 1980.

30. **Lee, S. H.,** Histochemical estrogen receptor assay, *Am. J. Clin. Pathol.,* 76, 365, 1981.

31. **Lee, S. H.,** Hydrophilic macromolecules of steroid derivatives for the detection of cancer cell receptors, *Cancer,* 46, 2825, 1980.

32. **Eriksson, H. A., Hardin, J. W., Markaverich, B., Upchurch, S., and Clark, J. H.,** Estrogen binding in the rat uterus: heterogeneity of sites and relation to uterotrophic response, *J. Steroid Biochem.,* 12, 121, 1980.

33. **Clark, J. H., Hardin, J. W., Upchurch, S., and Eriksson, H.,** Heterogeneity of estrogen binding sites in the cytosol of the rat uterus, *J. Biol. Chem.,* 253, 7630, 1978.

34. **Eriksson, H., Upchurch, S., Hardin, J. W., Peck, E. J., and Clark, J. H.,** Heterogeneity of estrogen receptors in the cytosol and nuclear fractions of the rat uterus, *Biochem. Biophys. Res. Commun.,* 81, 1, 1978.

35. **Clark, J. H., Anderson, J. N., and Peck, E. J.,** Estrogen receptor antiestrogen complex. Atypical binding by uterine nuclei and effects on uterine growth, *Steroids,* 22, 707, 1973.

36. **Murphy, L. C., Foo, M. S., Green, M. D., Milthorpe, B. K., Whybourne, A. M., Krozowski, Z. S., and Sutherland, R. L.,** Binding of non steroidal antioestrogens to saturable binding sites distinct from estrogen receptors in normal and neoplastic tissues, in *Program and Abstracts Antioestrogen Workshop,* Sydney, February 4 to 6, 1980.

37. **Markaverich, B. M. and Clark, J. H.,** Two binding sites for estradiol in rat uterine nuclei: relationship to uterotropic response, *Endocrinology,* 105, 1458, 1979.

38. **Russell, J., Newman, H. A. I., and Sharma, H. M.,** Histochemical estrogen receptor assay, *Am. J. Clin. Pathol.,* 75, 127, 1981.

39. **Pertschuk, L. P. and Gaetjens, E.,** Authors' reply, *Am. J. Clin. Pathol.,* 75, 128, 1981.

40. **Westfall, U., Ed.,** *Steroid Protein Interactions,* Springer-Verlag, Berlin, 1971.

41. **Rasmussen, B. B., Rose, C., Thorpe, S. M., Hou-Jensen, K., Daehnfeldt, J. L., and Palshof, T.,** Histo-pathological characteristics and oestrogen receptor content in primary breast carcinoma, *Virchows Arch. (Pathol. Anat.),* 390, 347, 1981.

42. **Hahnel, R.,** Steroid receptor status, tumour growth and prognosis, in *Endocrine Relationships in Breast Cancer,* Stoll, B. A., Ed., Heinemann, London, 1982, 107.

43. **Antoniades, K. and Spector, H.,** Correlation of estrogen receptor levels with histology and cytomorphology in human mammary cancer, *Am. J. Clin. Pathol.,* 71, 497, 1979.

44. **Mossler, J. E., McCarty, K. S., Woodard, B. J., Mitchener, L. M., and Johnston, W. W.,** Correlation of mean nuclear area with estrogen receptor content in aspiration cytology of breast carcinoma, *Acta Cytol.,* 26, 417, 1982.

45. **Baak, J. P. A. and Persijn, J.,** In search for the best qualitative microscopical or morphometrical predictor of oestrogen receptor in breast cancer, *Pathol. Res. Pract.,* 178, 307, 1984.

46. **Baak, J. P. A. and Oort, J., Eds.,** *A Manual of Morphometry in Diagnostic Pathology,* Springer-Verlag, Heidelberg, 1983.

47. **Korsten, C. B. and Persijn, J. P.,** Evaluation of and additional data of an improved simple charcoal method to determine estrogen receptors, *J. Clin. Chem. Clin. Biochem.,* 15, 297, 1977.

48. **Bloom, H. J. G.,** Prognosis in carcinoma of the breast, *Br. J. Cancer,* 4, 259, 1950.

49. **Bloom, H. J. G. and Richardson, W. W.,** Histological grading and prognosis in breast cancer, *Br. J. Cancer,* 2, 369, 1957.

50. **Scarff, R. W. and Torloni, H.,** Histological Typing of Breast Tumours, World Health Organization, Geneva, 1968, 19.

51. **Black, M. M. and Speer, F. D.,** Nuclear structure in cancer tissues, *Surg. Gynecol. Obstet.,* 105, 97, 1957.

52. **Baak, J. P. A., Kurver, P. H. J., de Snoo-Nieuwlaat, A. J. E., de Graaf, S., Makkink, B., and Boon, M. E.,** Prognostic indicators in breast cancer — morphometric methods, *Histopathology,* 6, 327, 1982.

53. **Cooley, W. W. and Lohnes, P. R., Eds.,** *Multivariate Data Analysis,* John Wiley & Sons, New York, 1971.

54. **Galen, R. S. and Gambino, S. R., Eds.,** *Beyond Normality: The Predictive Value and Efficiency of Medical Diagnosis,* John Wiley & Sons, New York, 1975, 10.

55. **Olszewski, W., Darzynkiewicz, Z., Rosen, P. P., Schwaitz, M. K., and Melamed, M. R.,** Flow cytometry of breast carcinoma. I. Relation of DNA ploidy level of histology and estrogen receptor, *Cancer,* 48, 980, 1981a.

56. **Olszewski, W., Darzynkiewicz, Z., Rosen, P. P., Schwaitz, M. K., and Melamed, M. R.,** Flow cytometry of breast carcinoma. II. Relation of tumor cell cycle distribution of histology and estrogen receptor, *Cancer,* 48, 985, 1981b.

57. **Meijer, J. S., Rao, B. R., Stevens, S. C., and White, W. L.,** Low incidence of estrogen receptor in breast carcinomas with rapid rates of cellular replication, *Cancer,* 40, 2290, 1977.

58. **Knight, W. A., Livingston, R. B., Gregory, E. J., and McGuire, W. L.,** Estrogen receptors as an independent prognostic factor for early recurrence in breast cancer, *Cancer Res.,* 37, 4669, 1977.

59. **Lippman, M. E. and Allegra, J. C.,** Quantitative estrogen receptor analysis. The response to endocrine and cytotoxic chemotherapy in human breast cancer and the disease free interval, *Cancer,* 46, 2829, 1980.

60. **McGuire, W. L., Chamness, G. C., Costlow, M. E., and Richert, N. J.,** Steroids and human breast cancer, *J. Steroid Biochem.,* 6, 723, 1975.

61. **Meijer, J. S., Stevens, S. C., White, W. L., and Hixon, B.,** Estrogen receptor assay of carcinoma of the breast by a simplified dextran charcoal method, *Am. J. Clin. Pathol.,* 70, 655, 1978.

62. **Pertschuk, L. P., Tobin, E. H., Brigati, D. J., Kim, D. S., Bloom, N. D., Gaetjens, E., Berman, P. J., Carter, A. C., and Degenshein, G. A.,** Immunofluorescent detection of estrogen receptors in breast cancer, *Cancer,* 41, 907, 1978.

63. **Jacobs, S. R., Wolfson, W. L., Cheng, L., and Lewin, K. J.,** Cytochemical and competitive protein binding assays for estrogen receptor in breast disease. A comparative study of 62 cases, *Cancer,* 51, 1621, 1983.

64. **Baak, J. P. A., Agrafojo Blanco, A., Kurver, P. H. J., Langley, F. A., Boon, M. E., Lindeman, J., Overdiep, S. H., Niewlaat, A., and Brekelmans, E.,** Quantitation of borderline and malignant mucinous ovarian tumors, *Histopathology,* 5, 353, 1981.

65. **McGuire, W. L., Horwitz, K. B., Zava, D. T., Carola, R. E., and Chamness, G. C.,** Hormones in breast cancer update, *Metabolism,* 27, 487, 1978.

66. **DeSombre, E. R. and Jensen, E. V.,** Estrophilin assays in breast cancer. Quantitative features and application to the mastectomy specimen, *Cancer,* 46, 2783, 1980.

67. **King, R. J. B.,** Quality control of estrogen receptor analysis. The United Kingdom experience, *Cancer,* 46, 2822, 1980.

68. **Paridaens, R., Sylvester, R. J., Ferrazzi, E., Legres, N., Leclercq, C., and Henson, J. C.,** Clinical significance of the quantitative assessment of estrogen receptors in advanced breast cancer, *Cancer,* 46, 2889, 1980.

69. **Underwood, J. C. E., Dangerfield, V. J. M., and Parsons, M. A.,** Oestrogen receptor assay of cryostat sections of human breast carcinomas with simultaneous quantitative histology, *J. Clin. Pathol.,* 36, 399, 1983.
70. **van Marle, J., Baak, J. P. A., Meijer, C. J. L. M., and Lindeman, J.,** unpublished results.

Chapter 9

# PEROXIDASE LABELING OF ESTROGEN BINDING SITES IN BREAST CANCER

**Rosemary A. Walker**

## TABLE OF CONTENTS

I.     Introduction ................................................................ 134

II.    Immunoperoxidase Studies .................................................. 134

III.   Histochemical Studies ...................................................... 135
       A.     Preparation of Peroxidase Conjugates ............................... 136
       B.     Tissue Preparation ................................................. 137
       C.     Staining Methods ................................................... 138
       D.     Staining Results ................................................... 139
       E.     Relationship to Morphology ......................................... 143
       F.     Correlation with Biochemical Assay ................................. 143

IV.    Conclusions ................................................................ 144

Acknowledgments ................................................................. 146

References ...................................................................... 146

# I. INTRODUCTION

Interest in the development of histological methods for assessment of the steroid binding capacity of human tumors has been for several reasons: their cheapness in terms of equipment and technician time and potential use in ordinary hospital laboratories; their ability to distinguish between normal and tumor tissue which cannot be achieved by biochemical methods that rely upon homogenization of tissue, with subsequent possible effects on their results; their potential for assessment of heterogeneity of expression of steroid binding within a tumor. The latter is of particular significance since the proportion of cells which have the capacity to bind steroids, compared to those which do not, may be an important factor in determining the endocrine responsiveness of an individual tumor.[1]

Many of the studies which have been concerned with histological techniques have utilized fluorescein, or other fluorescent agents, as a marker in both immunohistochemical[2-4] and histochemical methods.[5-9] The resulting preparations have the disadvantage of requiring an ultraviolet microscope for examination, and although they can be stored with care for a period of time they are not permanent. The assessment of the proportions of cells showing evidence of steroid binding and those not, one of the major attractions of histological methods, can be difficult, particularly to those not skilled in the interpretation of fluorescence. Cellular definition with respect to distinction between cytoplasm and nucleus can also cause problems.

It was because of these various difficulties that methods utilizing an enzyme as a label were used by the author.[10-12] Horseradish peroxidase was introduced as an alternative marker to fluorescein in immunohistochemistry in the 1960s.[15] Its advantages are that the histochemical method used to demonstrate the site of peroxidase within a section results in a permanent end product, which can be examined by an ordinary light microscope. Cellular definition is good, and distinction between cytoplasm and nucleus is assisted by the use of a nuclear counterstain. There can be problems, though, with using peroxidase as a marker in steroid binding studies and these will be discussed where relevant in the following sections.

The approaches available for the histological demonstration of steroid binding utilizing peroxidase are similar to those for fluorescein, namely, immunohistochemistry and histochemistry using enzyme-labeled hormone. These techniques will be discussed in some detail, as will the preparation of tissue which is the other important aspect of such histological methods.

# II. IMMUNOPEROXIDASE STUDIES

The immunofluorescent studies have used either monomeric estradiol[2] or polyestradiol phosphate;[3] similar approaches have been used for immunoperoxidase by some workers, but variations have been utilized particularly in studies on animal tissues. All methods rely on the use of an antiserum to estradiol and its subsequent localization by either peroxidase-labeled antiimmunoglobulin antiserum or antiimmunoglobulin antiserum and peroxidase-antiperoxidase complex.

Prebound endogenous estrogen has been detected in routinely fixed, paraffin-embedded sections of breast carcinomas from 10 out of 25 patients by Ghosh et al.,[14] using an antiserum to estradiol and peroxidase-antiperoxidase complex. Kurzon and Sternberger[15] studied estrogen binding in rat cervix; slices of tissue were incubated with 17β-estradiol before fixation in picric acid-formaldehyde, clearing, and embedding. They considered that the estradiol protected the specific binding sites during fixation but that was lost during embedding, since, unlike the previous study, there was no evidence of prebound estrogen. Staining was achieved when dewaxed tissue sections were incubated with estradiol prior to the application of antiserum to estradiol and the three-stage peroxidase-antiperoxidase complex method. This approach of incubation of tissue with estradiol prior to fixation and processing has not been applied to human breast carcinomas. Kopp et al.[16] have localized prebound estradiol in rat uterus in frozen sections, with fixation of the tissue after application of antiestradiol antiserum and prior to incubation with anti-rabbit immunoglobulin antiserum and peroxidase-antiperoxidase complex. They have extended the method to the ultrastructural level, which is an advantage of peroxidase over fluorescein.

Taylor et al.[17] examined human breast and endometrial carcinomas that had been routinely formalin-fixed, paraffin-embedded, using polyestradiol phosphate at a concentration of 1 mg/m$\ell$. This was followed, after fixation with 1% paraformaldehyde, by an antiserum to estradiol and the peroxidase-antiperoxidase complex method. A correlation with the biochemical dextran-coated charcoal method was found in 60% of cases. Mercer et al.[18] and Walker et al.[10] studied frozen sections of human breast carcinomas, incubating with monomeric estradiol at concentrations of $1 \times 10^{-7}$ and $5 \times 10^{-8}$ $M$, respectively, followed by antiserum to estradiol and peroxidase-labeled antiimmunoglobulin serum[18] or the peroxidase-antiperoxidase complex method.[10] Mercer et al. noted a reaction in 75% of cases with 71% consisting of varying proportions of positive and negative cells, but commented that from studies using MCF-7 cells, and in view of the high concentrations of estradiol required, it seemed unlikely that specific high-affinity receptors had been detected by this method. Walker et al. found only staining in a small proportion of cells in a few cases and considered that, since these findings were most likely unrepresentative of the hormone receptor status of the tumors, the method was unsuitable for the detection of steroid binding. Studies concerned with the abilities of antibodies to 17β-estradiol to recognize the hormone when receptor bound have concluded that they cannot.[19-21] Morrow et al.[21] studied polyestradiol phosphate, in particular, and considered that it interacted with nonspecific protein rather than high-affinity receptor protein, and that antiestradiol antibody could react with polyestradiol phosphate when complexed to these proteins. Underwood et al.[22] have suggested that the inaccessability of receptor-bound estradiol to estradiol antibodies is because the receptor-hormone interaction is of a clathrate type.

Besides the major problems that the concentration of estradiol required is higher than that defined for high-affinity specific binding,[23] and that antibodies to estradiol appear to be able to only detect nonspecific binding, the immunoperoxidase methods are rather cumbersome in that they require an extra step (i.e., incubation with estradiol) to the normal immunohistochemical procedure.

## III. HISTOCHEMICAL STUDIES

As an alternative to the immunohistochemical methods several studies have tried simpler approaches using either estradiol linked to fluorescein directly or through bovine serum albumin (BSA). Coupling has been at either the 6 or 17 position of estradiol. These variations can affect the efficiency of the conjugates in the histochemical procedures.

Theoretical considerations concerning the postulated site of the estradiol-receptor bond[24] would favor the 6 position as the site for coupling. Similarly, in the preparation of antisera to estradiol there is better preservation of antigenicity when the protein carrier is coupled at the 6 position.[25,26] However, Dandliker et al.[27] compared the relative binding affinities (RBA) for receptor of two conjugates in which fluorescein was directly coupled to the 6 or the 17 position, and found that the one for the latter was higher. A similar finding was reported by Penney and Hawkins.[28] This would suggest that conjugation through the 17 position is preferable for histochemical studies.

Barrows et al.[8] linked fluorescein through a succinamide-ethyl-amine chain to the 17 position of estradiol, which resulted in a conjugate of relatively low molecular weight and with a reasonable RBA.[23] Penney and Hawkins[28] considered the effect of using BSA as a link in conjugates in relation to the RBA and found a much lower level for 17β-estradiol-

BSA-fluorescein prepared by themselves than that found for the above direct-linked conjugate. They also assessed the estradiol-BSA-fluorescein conjugate prepared by Pertschuk et al.[7] and found that it had a much higher RBA, but could not exclude the effect of free estradiol, due to degradation, in the sample.

It would, therefore, seem that the use of simple, direct-labeled estradiol conjugates would be preferable with regard to better tissue penetration due to low molecular weight, size, and affinity for receptor. However, the methods available for the conjugation of enzymes such as horseradish peroxidase all involve linkage to a protein. The use of an estradiol-BSA complex, is, therefore, necessary, so resulting in the formation of a large molecular weight compound. This is one of the disadvantages of peroxidase over fluorescein.

## A. Preparation of Peroxidase Conjugates

In the studies undertaken by the author[10-12] the estradiol-BSA complex has been obtained commercially in the form 17β-estradiol-6-*O*-carboxy methyloxime-bovine serum albumin from both Uniscience and Steraloids. More recently 17β-estradiol 17β-hemisuccinate-bovine serum albumin has been obtained from Sigma. Gaetjens and Pertschuk[29] have described a modification of the previously reported method[30] for the coupling of albumin to steroids.

The most widely used methods for the conjugation of horseradish peroxidase are the two-stage glutaraldehyde technique of Avrameas and Ternynck[31] and the periodate method of Nakane and Kawaoi.[32] Both have been used in the preparation of estradiol-BSA-peroxidase conjugates. The glutaraldehyde method relies on the differing reactivities of two proteins towards glutaraldehyde, which acts as a bifunctional coupling reagent; horseradish peroxidase is rather unreactive due to the paucity of free amino groups in the protein molecule. The periodate method is a two-stage coupling reaction in which a reactive functional group is generated in peroxidase by oxidation of carbohydrate moieties with the periodate. A modification of the latter method, in which the need for reagents to block horseradish peroxidase self-coupling is eliminated, has been described.[33]

Separation of free estradiol-BSA from that labeled by the conjugation procedure has been undertaken by column chromatography with Sephadex® G100 (Pharmacia).[11] Boorsma and Streefkerk[34] have suggested that polyacrylamide-agarose is preferable to dextran gels such as Sepharose for the separation of peroxidase conjugates. Another approach is affinity chromatography. Concanavalin A has a high affinity for mannose, which is a component of horseradish peroxidase, so this lectin, when coupled to a gel such as Sepharose 4B, can be utilized to separate peroxidase conjugates from unlabeled substances.[35] This is illustrated in Figure 1 in which the first peak consists of estradiol-BSA and the second peak estradiol-BSA-peroxidase plus free peroxidase, which have been eluted from the column of Concanavalin A-Sepharose 4B by the addition of a gradient of α-methyl-D-mannoside.

Analysis of the efficiency of the binding of horseradish peroxidase to estradiol-BSA with the two methods of conjugation has shown that the periodate method has resulted in 50% binding in some instances and up to 70% binding on other occasions, whereas the binding achieved with the glutaraldehyde method has been more consistent but lower at 7.5% peroxidase and 25% estradiol-BSA.[12] These figures are similar to those found for the coupling of peroxidase to antibodies.[36]

Although the periodate method results in a greater degree of binding between peroxidase and estradiol-BSA, higher concentrations of the conjugates prepared in this way are required to achieve staining than compared with glutaraldehyde-prepared conjugates (see "Staining Methods"). There have been similar findings for peroxidase-labeled antibody prepared by the periodate method compared to that prepared by the glutaraldehyde method,[37] and this has been thought to be due to the formation of high molecular weight polymeric conjugates with the periodate procedure which have poorer penetration of tissue sections. The same study has shown that there is a greater degree of inhibition of enzyme activity with the

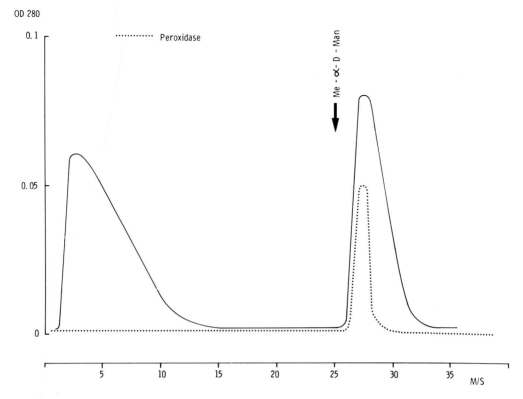

FIGURE 1. The separation of unlabeled estradiol-BSA (first peak) from estradiol-BSA-peroxidase (second peak) by the use of Concanavalin A-Sepharose 4B. The conjugate is eluted by the addition of α-methyl-D-mannoside and the volume is in milliliters.

periodate method than the glutaraldehyde method, and, also, that there is loss of binding activity of the coupled protein which does not occur with fluorescein conjugation. This is one of the other disadvantages of using peroxidase rather than fluorescein for the histochemical detection of estrogen binding, and is probably one of the factors determining the low RBA found for the estradiol-BSA-peroxidase conjugate by Penney and Hawkins.[28]

These studies indicate that although the yield from the glutaraldehyde method is low the formation of essentially monomeric complexes for histological studies is preferable to the polymeric complexes formed with the periodate conjugation procedure.

## B. Tissue Preparation

The major problems concerned with the preparation of tissue for the histological detection of estrogen binding relate to the receptor, which is a soluble protein and, therefore, subject to extraction in aqueous media.[38]

Although Taylor et al.[17] suggest that estrogen binding can be detected in routinely processed formalin-fixed, paraffin-embedded tissue, this has not been the finding of the author.[10-12] The use of tissue frozen by a method that facilitates rapid freezing, such as isopentane precooled in liquid nitrogen, within 30 min of excision from the patient, appears to be essential.[11] The length of storage time before examination of tissue is also important, since results with material stored beyond 2 months can be variable. Reexamination of the same blocks of tissue also results in a deterioration in staining, presumably due to thawing, then refreezing.

Sections (6 to 8 μm) are cut in a cryostat at −20°C from the frozen tissue and mounted on chemically clean slides. They are then air-dried at room temperature for 2 to 3 min or treated with acetone, also at room temperature, for the same period of time. This is allowed to evaporate before application of the conjugate. A variety of air-drying and fixation procedures have been assessed.[11] These show that longer periods of air-drying, whether at 4°C or room temperature, result in diffusion of staining with decreased or absent cell reaction; exposure to acetone for more than 5 min leads to loss of staining; the use of alcohol results in a fine granular staining of tissue stroma rather than cells; and that there is an absence of reaction after treatment with 4% formaldehyde in saline for any period of time.

The effect on estrogen receptor activity of tissue sectioning and exposure to aqueous media with and without fixation has been assessed by Penney and Hawkins.[28] They found that receptor activity is very readily lost from unfixed tissues into the media, that acetone fixation appears to destroy at least 50% of receptor, and that fixation with agents such as ethanol/acetone after incubation[7] abolishes steroid binding. From their studies it would appear that the method using brief fixation of frozen sections by acetone might allow some 25% of estrogen receptor originally in the tissue to remain viable. Although this is not an ideal situation the preparation of tissue by this method would seem, from the simple histochemical studies and more sophisticated assessment of receptor activity, to be the most appropriate one.

## C. Staining Methods

Tissue sections are prepared as described above and incubated with estradiol-BSA-peroxidase in a Perspex box having a moist atmosphere for 2 hr at room temperature. They are then rinsed and washed in Tris-saline buffer (pH 7.6) for 15 min. The peroxidase is localized by the diaminobenzidine-hydrogen peroxide reaction[39] with a resultant brown color. Nuclei are counterstained by brief exposure to Mayer's hemalum, then the sections are dehydrated, cleared, and mounted. Two or three blocks of tissue are assessed for each case.

The concentrations of conjugates used for staining have varied depending on the method of peroxidase coupling involved. For the periodate-prepared conjugates concentrations have ranged from 125 µg/mℓ ($5 \times 10^{-7}$ M estradiol) to 268 µg/mℓ ($1 \times 10^{-6}$ M estradiol), whereas for glutaraldehyde-prepared conjugates it has been 60 µg/mℓ ($2 \times 10^{-7}$ M estradiol). These are for the conjugates in which BSA is coupled through the 6 position. A recently prepared conjugate in which the coupling of BSA is through the 17 position has been used at a concentration of 30 µg/mℓ ($1 \times 10^{-7}$ M estradiol). The main problem with this conjugate is related to the relative insolubility of the 17β-estradiol 17 hemisuccinate-BSA resulting in an inefficient coupling of peroxidase.

The major competitive controls for staining are the prior and coincubation of sections with 100 times excess tamoxifen (ICI) and diethylstilbestrol. Other controls are the use of BSA-peroxidase in place of estradiol-BSA-peroxidase and the diaminobenzidine-hydrogen peroxide reaction alone to detect endogenous peroxidase. Other tissues have been examined, namely, lung, stomach, and tonsil, to act as negative controls. Cytospin preparations of MCF-7 breast carcinoma cells, which are known to possess estrogen receptors, have also been stained. Samples from breast tissue considered to be normal or showing hyperplastic change have been examined in the same manner as tissue from breast carcinomas. Competition for binding by the coincubation with excess progesterone has also been undertaken on several occasions.

The method of assessment is based on calculating the percentage of cells showing a positive reaction in 30 random high-power fields for each sample from all cases. Variation in intensity of staining within an individual section is considered but not between sections.

It can be seen that the concentrations of estradiol required to achieve staining fall outside that at which saturation of high-affinity estrogen receptors is achieved ($10^{-9}$ M). This has been one of the major criticisms of the histochemical methods.[23] A second, specific estrogen binding site (named type II as opposed to the high-affinity type I) has been demonstrated

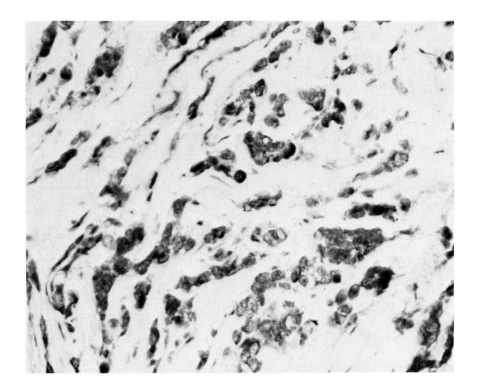

FIGURE 2.  Breast carcinoma with many cells having evidence of estrogen binding, there being a clearly definable reaction and no background staining. (Estradiol-BSA-peroxidase; magnification × 160.)

in human breast carcinomas.[40] It has a lower affinity for estrogen and is present in higher concentrations than the classical cytoplasmic estrogen receptor. It would, therefore, seem that with the concentrations of estradiol-BSA-peroxidase being used in the histochemical method that it is this type II binding site that is being demonstrated. Estrogen binding can also occur to albumin and other soluble molecules and is probably a factor if still higher concentrations of estrogen are used.[23]

## D. Staining Results

The histochemical reaction for peroxidase results in a clearly definable brown end product, which contrasts with the light blue of nuclei. There is no loss of staining intensity with time and all preparations can be examined by an ordinary light microscope. Figure 2 is of a carcinoma in which many of the cells gave a positive reaction and illustrates the contrast between the cells and the background connective tissue of which there is no staining. The assessment of percentage cell binding is, thus, easy in such preparations.

Examination of tissue sections from samples of normal or hyperplastic breast tissue has shown staining of essentially all cells, but with variation of intensity of reaction within individual cases. The numbers of positive cells within carcinomas has ranged from 20 to 85%. Variation between samples from the same tumor has been up to 15%, but there have been no instances of one section having many positive cells and another from the same case having few. There has been no evidence of staining of any of the cells of tumors that have been negative.

The distribution of staining in those carcinomas not having the majority of cells reacting has been as groups of positive cells of varying sizes throughout the sections, with no evidence

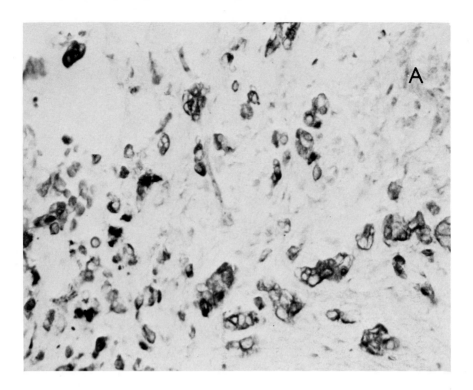

FIGURE 3.    Breast carcinoma with 60% of cells staining. There is one group of negative cells (labeled A), but individual negative cells can be seen between the positive ones. (Estradiol-BSA-peroxidase; magnification × 160.)

of clustering, in contrast to the staining pattern seen in the immunohistochemical localization of some tumor markers.[41] Figures 3 to 5 illustrate the appearances seen dependent upon the number of cells reacting. In Figure 3, although there is one larger group of negative cells, individual and small groups of cells lacking a reaction can be seen intermingled with positive cells. The juxtaposition of positive and negative cells is clearly seen in Figure 4, and in Figure 5 only small numbers of cells react, and these show a variation in staining intensity.

The reaction can be identified in the cytoplasm and/or nucleus of cells. It is because of the nuclear staining that it is essential that there is only a brief counterstaining with hematoxylin. A group of cells having both cytoplasmic and nuclear staining is shown in Figure 6, and nuclear staining alone in Figure 7. The cytoplasmic reaction has been predominantly a diffuse one, with occasionally an accentuation at the cell periphery or in the perinuclear region. Staining in the nucleus appears to be in relation to chromatin and, in some instances, the nucleolus has been the main site of reaction. A small number of tumors (6%) shows nuclear staining only; this figure is similar to that found with fluorescent conjugates.[42] The significance of this nuclear reaction is difficult to evaluate when a ''static'' histochemical procedure is used. Lee[6] has tended to disregard it. Pertschuk et al.[42] have found that patients whose tumors showed nuclear staining alone had a poor therapeutic response to hormonal therapy. In several studies translocation of estrogen binding sites from cytoplasm to nucleus has been demonstrated in either cell suspensions by immunofluorescence[2,43] or in tissue sections with fluorescent conjugates.[8,44] It is uncertain whether the nuclear staining detected in this study represents nuclear translocation, which is unlikely in view of the clinical finding of Pertschuk, or is a separate nuclear binding site.

The treatment of control sections with tamoxifen or diethylstilbestrol, either prior to the

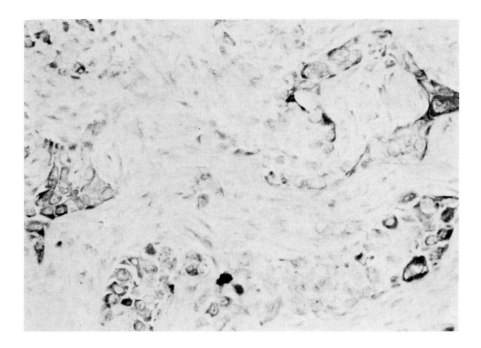

FIGURE 4. Breast carcinoma with 30% of cells staining. Positive and negative cells can be seen adjacent to one another. (Estradiol-BSA-peroxidase; magnification × 160.)

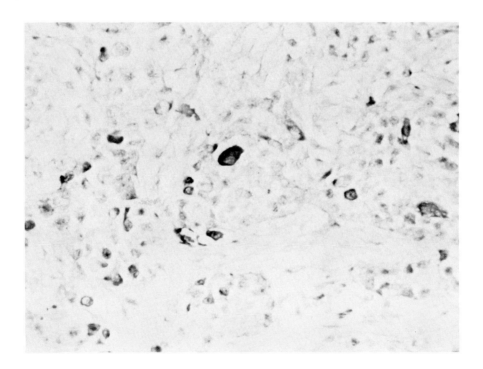

FIGURE 5. Breast carcinoma with 20% of cells reacting. Single positive cells can be seen throughout and there is some variation in intensity. (Estradiol-BSA-peroxidase; magnification × 160.)

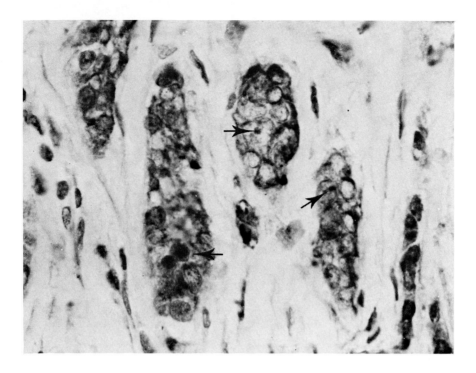

FIGURE 6.   Groups of positive cells which show both staining of cytoplasm and nucleus (arrowed). (Estradiol-BSA-peroxidase; magnification × 480.)

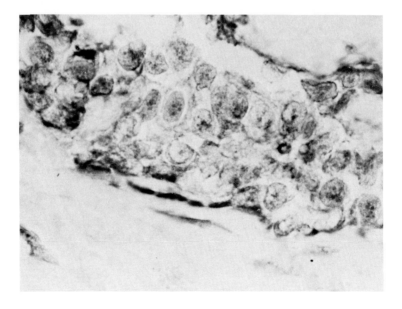

FIGURE 7.   Essentially only nuclear staining of chromatin in a group of breast carcinoma cells. (Estradiol-BSA-peroxidase; magnification × 480.)

application of estradiol-BSA-peroxidase or as a coincubation, has resulted in a lack of staining, indicating that the binding of the conjugate is to specific sites. However, this type of control will not differentiate between binding to type I or type II sites. Penney and Hawkins[28] experienced difficulty in achieving blocking of staining by estradiol-BSA-peroxidase with unlabeled competitors and noted that the latter had to be used as a saturated solution. No reaction has been seen when BSA-peroxidase alone has been used. Endogeneous peroxidase has never been identified in breast carcinoma cells. Sections of lung, stomach, and tonsil have consistently shown no evidence of estrogen binding, whereas MCF-7 cells have exhibited staining, although with some variation between cells, whenever examined. On the instances when competition by a nonestrogenic agent has been undertaken there has been no alteration of estrogen binding.

### E. Relationship to Morphology

All cases of intraduct carcinoma examined have shown evidence of estrogen binding, as have mucinous and infiltrating lobular carcinomas. The percentage of cells staining in the latter tumors has been quite low in some instances. Of the infiltrating duct carcinomas assessed, 74% (89/120) have given a positive reaction.

All carcinomas that have been investigated have had the degree of histological differentiation assessed by the use of the grading criteria of Bloom and Richardson,[45] with a modification in that only mitotic figures and not mitotic figures plus hyperchromatic nuclei were considered in that category. Hematoxylin and eosin stained sections from two blocks of paraffin-processed tumor tissue have been examined. The correlation between the degree of differentiation, divided into grades I, well differentiated, II, moderately differentiated, and III, poorly differentiated and the degree of estrogen binding (negative or percentage of positive cells) is shown in Figure 8. It can be seen that all of the well-differentiated carcinomas have given a positive reaction and that in all instances more than 50% of cells have stained. The moderately differentiated tumors exhibit heterogeneity, with 13% being negative, 18.5% having less than 50% of positive cells, and 68.5% more than 50% reactive cells. In contrast 67% of the poorly differentiated carcinomas have been negative, 18% have less than 50% cells reacting, and only 15% have more than 50% of cells positive. This striking relationship between estrogen binding and histological differentiation has also been noted for biochemical assays.[46,47]

### F. Correlation with Biochemical Assay

Eighty carcinomas which have been examined by the histochemical method have also been assessed by the dextran-coated charcoal assay.[10-12] Sixty-three (80%) have given a positive reaction with the histological technique; a further 55 tumors tested but without biochemical correlation have shown staining in 73%; 70% of carcinomas have had estrogen receptor detectable by the biochemical assay, and all of these have been positive by the histochemical method. There has been a correlation between the two methods in 91% of cases, a finding similar to that of Pertschuk et al.[7] Of those carcinomas that have given a positive reaction with the histological method alone, four have shown nuclear staining only, one has been an infiltrating lobular carcinoma with few neoplastic cells in a dense stroma, and two have been intraduct carcinomas, in whom sampling may have been a problem.

Penney and Hawkins[28] compared histochemical with biochemical assays and considered that since blocking of the conjugate could not be demonstrable in many of the cases, a correlation could only be found in 6 out of 25 assays.

The relationship between receptor concentration per milligram cytosol protein as assessed by the dextran-coated charcoal method and the percentage of positive cells was initially reported for 35 carcinomas;[10] a poor quantitative correlation was noted. Extension of the findings to 80 carcinomas confirms this result (Figure 9). Those tumors with 80% of cells

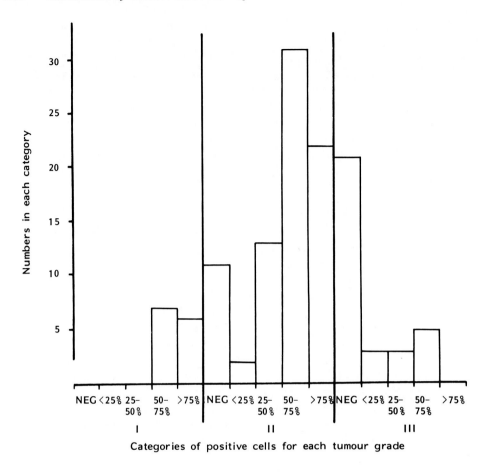

FIGURE 8.    The numbers of carcinomas giving a particular reaction for each tumor grade.

positive have shown a range from 10 to 450 fmol/mg cytosol protein on biochemical assay. The histochemical method only considers one aspect, i.e., the numbers of cells having a reaction, whereas the biochemical procedures will incorporate both numbers and the amount per cell, but this cannot alone account for such a wide variation.

There is at present insufficient clinical data, the studies having been performed prospectively on tumors from stage I and stage II patients, to assess the usefulness of the histochemical assays in determining clinical response to hormone therapy. It is with this approach that the best assessment of histological methods can be made, in particular, the significance of the heterogeneity of reaction which is so apparent with these techniques.

## IV. CONCLUSIONS

Peroxidase-labeled estradiol-BSA conjugates can be used to assess steroid binding in breast carcinomas, although with the range of concentrations used it is likely that it is type II binding sites that are detected. Clearly definable stable preparations are obtained which can easily be assessed with a standard light microscope. Of the two methods described for the conjugation of peroxidase, the two-stage glutaraldehyde one is to be preferred, since although the coupling is less efficient it results in monomeric complexes, whereas the periodate method leads to the formation of polymeric complexes with poorer capacity for tissue penetration. One of the major problems with the histological methods for assessment

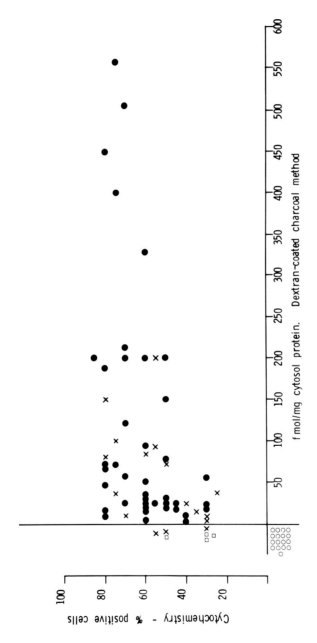

FIGURE 9.    Correlation between the percentage of cells reacting by the histochemical method, with the staining pattern, and the concentration of estrogen receptor as assessed by biochemical assay. ○ — Negative, □ — nuclear staining only, × — cytoplasmic staining only, ● — cytoplasmic and nuclear staining.

of steroid binding is the preparation of the tissue. The use of brief fixation of frozen sections in acetone would seem to be a reasonable compromise. Blocking of staining by the competitors tamoxifen and diethylstilbestrol has been achieved.

A good qualitative correlation has been demonstrated with the dextran-coated charcoal assay, but a poor quantitative one. A striking feature of the histological method, which is easily assessed with peroxidase preparations, is the cellular heterogeneity of binding within breast carcinomas, and this may be of clinical importance with regard to hormone therapy.

## ACKNOWLEDGMENTS

I am grateful to Drs. D. H. Cove, A. Howell, A. Hughes, Mrs. G. Barker, and Miss A. O'Toole for the biochemical estimations of estrogen receptor; Mrs. G. Holmes for typing the manuscript; and Ms. B. Jordan for photographic assistance.

## REFERENCES

1. **DeSombre, E. R., Greene, G. L., and Jensen, E. V.,** Estrophilin and endocrine responsiveness of breast cancer, in *Hormones Receptors and Breast Cancer,* McGuire, W. L., Ed., Raven Press, New York, 1978, chap. 1.
2. **Nenci, I., Beccati, M. D., Piffanelli, A., and Lanza, G.,** Detection and dynamic localization of oestradiol-receptor complexes in intact target cells by immunofluorescent technique, *J. Steroid Biochem.,* 7, 505, 1976.
3. **Pertschuk, L. P., Tobin, E. H., Brigati, D. J., Kim, D. S., Bloom, N. D., Gaetjens, E., Berman, P. J., Carter, A. C., and Degenshein, G. A.,** Immunofluorescent detection of estrogen receptors in breast cancer: comparison with dextran-coated charcoal and sucrose gradient assays, *Cancer,* 41, 907, 1978.
4. **Mercer, W. D., Carlson, C. A., Wahl, T. M., and Teague, P. O.,** Identification of estrogen receptors in mammary cancer cells by immunofluorescence, *Am. J. Clin. Pathol.,* 70, 330, 1978.
5. **Lee, S. H.,** Cytochemical study of estrogen receptor in human mammary cancer, *Am. J. Clin. Pathol.,* 70, 197, 1978.
6. **Lee, S. H.,** Cancer cell estrogen receptor of human mammary carcinoma, *Cancer,* 44, 1, 1979.
7. **Pertschuk, L. P., Gaetjens, E., Carter, A. C., Brigati, D. J., Kim, D. S., and Fealey, T. E.,** An improved histochemical method for the detection of estrogen receptors in mammary carcinoma, *Am. J. Clin. Pathol.,* 71, 504, 1979.
8. **Barrows, G. H., Stroupe, S. B., and Riehm, J. D.,** Nuclear uptake of ethyl-succinamide bridged 17β estradiol-fluorescein as a marker of estrogen receptor activity, *Am. J. Clin. Pathol.,* 73, 330, 1980.
9. **Nenci, I., Dandliker, W. B., Meyers, C. Y., Marchetti, E., Mazola, A., and Fabris, G.,** Estrogen receptor cytochemistry by fluorescent oestrogen, *J. Histochem. Cytochem.,* 28, 1081, 1980.
10. **Walker, R. A., Cove, D. H., and Howell, A.,** Histological detection of oestrogen receptor in human breast carcinomas, *Lancet,* 1, 171, 1980.
11. **Walker, R. A.,** The cytochemical demonstration of oestrogen receptors in human breast carcinomas, *J. Pathol.,* 135, 237, 1981.
12. **Walker, R. A.,** The use of peroxidase-labelled hormones in the study of steroid binding in breast carcinomas, in *Proc. 11th Int. Congr. of Clinical Chemistry,* Kaiser, E., Gabl, F., Mueller, M. H., and Bayer, M., Eds., Walter de Gruyter, Berlin, 1982, 507.
13. **Nakane, P. K. and Pierce, G. B., Jr.,** Enzymes labelled antibodies: preparation and application for localisation of antigens, *J. Histochem. Cytochem.,* 14, 929, 1966.
14. **Ghosh, L., Ghosh, B. C., and Das Gupta, T. K.,** Immunocytological localisation of estrogen in human mammary carcinoma cells by horseradish-anti-horseradish peroxidase complex, *J. Surg. Oncol.,* 10, 221, 1978.
15. **Kurzon, R. M. and Sternberger, L. A.,** Estrogen receptor immunocytochemistry, *J. Histochem. Cytochem.,* 26, 803, 1978.
16. **Kopp, F., Martin, P. M., Rolland, P. H., and Bertrand, F.-F.,** A preliminary report on the use of immunoperoxidases to study binding of estrogens in rat uteri, *J. Steroid Biochem.,* 11, 1081, 1979.

17. **Taylor, C. R., Cooper, C. L., Kurman, R. J., Goebelsmann, U., and Markland, F. S.,** Detection of estrogen receptor in breast and endometrial carcinoma by the immunoperoxidase technique, *Cancer,* 47, 2634, 1981.

18. **Mercer, W. D., Lippman, M. E., Wahl, T. M., Carlson, C. A., Wahl, D. A., Lezotte, D., and Teague, P. O.,** The use of immunocytochemical techniques for the detection of steroid hormones in breast cancer cells, *Cancer,* 46, 2859, 1980.

19. **Fishman, J. and Fishman, J. H.,** Competitive binding assay for estradiol receptor using immobilized antibody, *J. Clin. Endocrinol. Metab.,* 39, 603, 1974.

20. **Casteneda, E. and Liao, S.,** The use of anti-steroid antibodies in the characterisation of steroid receptors, *J. Biol. Chem.,* 250, 883, 1975.

21. **Morrow, B., Leav, I., DeLellis, R. A., and Raam, S.,** Use of polyestradiol phosphate and anti-17β estradiol antibodies for the localisation of estrogen receptor in target tissues: a critique, *Cancer,* 46, 2872, 1980.

22. **Underwood, J. C. E., Sher, E., Reed, M., Eisman, J. A., and Martin, T. J.,** Biochemical assessment of histochemical methods for oestrogen receptor localisation, *J. Clin. Pathol.,* 35, 401, 1982.

23. **Chamness, G. C., Mercer, W. D., and McGuire, W. L.,** Are histochemical methods for estrogen receptor valid?, *J. Histochem. Cytochem.,* 28, 792, 1980.

24. **Ellis, D. J. and Ringold, H. J.,** The uterine oestrogen receptor: a physiochemical study, in *The Sex Steroids,* McKerns, K. W., Ed., Appleton-Century-Crofts, New York, 1971, chap. 3.

25. **Exley, D., Johnson, M. W., and Dean, P. D. G.,** Antisera highly specific for 17-estradiol, *Steroids,* 18, 605, 1971.

26. **Lindner, H. R., Perel, E., Friedlander, A., and Zeitlin, A.,** Specificity of antibodies to ovarian hormones in relation to the site of attachment of the steroid hapten to the peptide carrier, *Steroids,* 19, 357, 1972.

27. **Dandliker, W. B., Brawn, R. J., Hsu, M.-L., Brawn, P. N., Levin, J., Meyers, C. Y., and Kolb, V. M.,** Investigation of hormone-receptor interactions by means of fluorescent labelling, *Cancer Res.,* 38, 4212, 1978.

28. **Penney, G. C. and Hawkins, R. A.,** Histochemical detection of oestrogen receptor: a progress report, *Br. J. Cancer,* 45, 237, 1982.

29. **Gaetjens, E. and Pertschuk, L. P.,** Synthesis of fluorescein labelled steroid hormone-albumin conjugates for the fluorescent histochemical detection of hormone receptors, *J. Steroid Biochem.,* 13, 1001, 1980.

30. **Erlanger, B. F., Borek, F., Beiser, S. M., and Leiberman, S.,** Preparation and characterisation of conjugates of bovine serum albumin with testosterone and with cortisone, *J. Biol. Chem.,* 228, 713, 1959.

31. **Avrameas, S. and Ternynck, T.,** Peroxidase labelled antibody and Fab conjugates with enhanced intracellular penetration, *Immunochemistry,* 8, 1175, 1971.

32. **Nakane, P. K. and Kawaoi, A.,** Peroxidase-labelled antibody a new method of conjugation, *J. Histochem. Cytochem.,* 22, 1084, 1974.

33. **Wilson, M. B. and Nakane, P. K.,** Recent developments in the periodate method of conjugating horseradish peroxidase (HRPO) to antibodies, in *Immunofluorescence and Related Staining Techniques,* Knapp, W., Holubar, K., and Wicks, G., Eds., Elsevier/North-Holland, Amsterdam, 1978, 215.

34. **Boorsma, D. M. and Streefkerk, J. G.,** Peroxidase-conjugate chromatography. Isolation of conjugates prepared with glutaraldehyde or periodate using polyacrylamide-agarose gel, *J. Histochem. Cytochem.,* 24, 481, 1976.

35. **Boorsma, D. M. and Steefkerk, J. G.,** Improved method for separation of peroxidase conjugates, in *Immunofluorescence and Related Staining Techniques,* Knapp, W., Holubar, K., and Wick, G., Eds., Elsevier/North-Holland, Amsterdam, 1978, 225.

36. **Boorsma, D. M. and Streefkerk, J. G.,** Some aspects of the preparation, analysis and use of peroxidase-antibody conjugates in immunohistochemistry, *Protides Biol. Fluids,* 24, 795, 1976.

37. **Boorsma, D. M., Streefkerk, J. G., and Kors, N.,** Peroxidase and fluorescein isothiocyanate as antibody markers. A quantitative comparison of two peroxidase conjugates prepared with glutaraldehyde or periodate and a fluorescein conjugate, *J. Histochem. Cytochem.,* 24, 1017, 1976.

38. **McCarty, K. S., Jr., Woodward, B. H., Nichols, D. E., Wilkinson, W., and McCarty, K. S., Sr.,** Comparison of biochemical and histochemical techniques of estrogen receptor analyses in mammary carcinoma, *Cancer,* 46, 2842, 1980.

39. **Graham, R. C. and Karnowsky, M. J.,** The early stages of absorption of injected horseradish peroxidase in the proximal tubules of mouse kidney; ultrastructural cytochemistry by a new technique, *J. Histochem. Cytochem.,* 14, 291, 1966.

40. **Panko, W. B., Watson, C. S., and Clark, J. H.,** The presence of a second, specific estrogen binding site in human breast cancer, *J. Steroid Biochem.,* 14, 1311, 1981.

41. **Walker, R. A.,** Significance of α-subunit HCG demonstrated in breast carcinomas by the immunoperoxidase technique, *J. Clin. Pathol.,* 31, 245, 1978.

42. **Pertschuk, L. P., Tobin, E. H., Tanapat, P., Gaetjens, E., Carter, A. C., Bloom, N. D., Macchia, R. J., and Eisenberg, K. B.,** Histochemical analyses of steroid hormone receptors in breast and prostatic carcinoma, *J. Histochem. Cytochem.,* 28, 799, 1980.

43. **Nenci, I.,** Receptor and centriole pathways of steroid action in normal and neoplastic cells, *Cancer Res.,* 38, 4204, 1978.

44. **Pertschuk, L. P., Gaetjens, E., Carter, A. C., and Macchia, R. J.,** Histochemical detection of estrogen receptor (ER) translocation in breast and prostatic tumours, *Fed. Proc.,* 39, 414, 1980.

45. **Bloom, H. J. G. and Richardson, W. W.,** Histological grading and prognosis in breast cancer, *Br. J. Cancer,* 11, 359, 1957.

46. **Maynard, P. V., Davies, C. J., Blamey, R. W., Elston, C. N., Johnson, J., and Griffiths, K.,** Relationship between oestrogen-receptor content and histological grade in primary breast tumours, *Br. J. Cancer,* 38, 745, 1978.

47. **McCarty, K. S., Jr., Barton, T. K., Fetter, B. F., Woodard, B. H., Mossler, J. A., Reeves, W., Daly, J., Wilkinson, W. E., and McCarty, K. S., Sr.,** Correlation of estrogen and progesterone receptors with histologic differentiation in mammary carcinoma, *Cancer,* 46, 2851, 1980.

Chapter 10

# CRITICAL ISSUES IN THE EVALUATION OF HISTOCHEMICAL AND BIOCHEMICAL METHODS FOR STEROID RECEPTOR ANALYSIS*

**Kenneth S. McCarty, Jr., David L. Ingram, and Kenneth S. McCarty, Sr.**

## TABLE OF CONTENTS

I.      Introduction ................................................................. 150

II.     Brief History ............................................................... 150

III.    Data Acquisition and Analysis .............................................. 150

IV.     Biochemical Evaluation of the Estrogen Receptor ........................... 151
        A.      Methods ........................................................... 151
        B.      Biochemical Characteristics of ER ................................. 152
        C.      Limitations ....................................................... 153
        D.      Clinical Correlations ............................................. 154

V.      Histologic Correlations with ER ........................................... 154
        A.      Tumor Type ........................................................ 154
        B.      Tumor Grade ....................................................... 155
        C.      Other Histologic Features ......................................... 155

VI.     Histologic Correlation with Other Substances .............................. 155

VII.    Histochemistry ............................................................ 156
        A.      Considerations .................................................... 156
        B.      Methods ........................................................... 157
                1.      Ligand-Antibody Method ................................... 157
                2.      Labeled Ligand Method .................................... 158
        C.      Receptor-Antibody Methods ......................................... 158

References ...................................................................... 159

* This work was supported in part by: NCI-2P30-CA-14236-11A1; NCI-2PO1-CA-11265-14; NCI-5RO1-CA-28720-03; and NCI-1PO1-CA-32672-02.

# I. INTRODUCTION

The presence of sex steroid receptors in human carcinomas was first convincingly shown by Jensen and co-workers in the 1960s.[1-3] Subsequently, the clinical value of assessing the presence of estrogen binding proteins in tumor tissues was studied by many investigators. As a consequence of these studies, assays for estrogen receptor (ER) have become an indispensible element in the evaluation of patients with malignant breast tumors. Constraints on the tumor volume of tissue required for multiconcentration ligand binding analysis as well as issues of "tumor heterogeneity" have led to an exploration of alternative methods for evaluating ER content. Thus, the promise of a simple, inexpensive, and rapid method of assessing ER content in histologic sections of breast tumor by histochemical or immunohistochemical analysis has attracted a great deal of attention. Several approaches using various labeling techniques have been used in an attempt to establish a valid and reproducible histochemical method to evaluate tissue steroid receptor content. While it is apparent that some of the problems associated with the biochemical assay may be resolved by histochemistry, a new set of problems arises, emphasizing that each approach must be rigorously tested in its own right. The various histochemical techniques reported to date are discussed and compared to what is known regarding the capacity of these procedures to adequately evaluate ER *in situ* or otherwise.

# II. BRIEF HISTORY

The pioneering report by Beatson in 1896 which demonstrated the response of certain breast carcinomas to hormonal manipulation was an empirical observation preceding by 60 years the discovery of steroid receptor proteins.[4] On the basis of Beatson's observations, ablation of the ovaries by surgery or radiation represented the preferred therapy of advanced breast cancer. Subsequently, it was observed that with the alternatives of oophorectomy, adrenalectomy, and hypophysectomy, the response rate for patients with metastatic breast cancer treated by endocrine ablation was approximately 30%.[5,6] The selection of patients for whom these therapeutic procedures were being used had been derived from empirical observations relating to the clinical course of disease and menopausal status of the patient. However, in 1960 Jensen et al.[1] described the binding of labeled estrogen in the reproductive target tissues of animal models. Folca et al.,[2] in 1961, showed increased binding in vivo of an estrogen derivative in hormonally responsive tumors as compared with unresponsive lesions. Extraction of a high-affinity binding protein was then accomplished by Toft and Gorski.[3] Shortly thereafter Jensen et al.[7] reported the presence of such estrogen receptors in certain human mammary carcinomas. These studies led to the hypothesis that ER-positive tumors would exhibit increased hormonal response over ER-negative tumors, a concept which has since been confirmed independently by numerous studies.[8-11] Published clinical trials which have shown the clinical utility of estrogen receptor determinations have each emphasized the importance of quantitation of the number of binding sites, the dissociation constant of the binding ($K_d$), and the physical parameters of the receptor proteins.

# III. DATA ACQUISITION AND ANALYSIS

In the testing of methods to evaluate ER content, as in any analytic procedure, it is important to adhere to certain guidelines that establish its validity and accuracy.[12] One of the critical and essential elements is the definition of the criteria by which experimental observations will be judged. For example, true positive results may be defined in relation to: (1) a biologic response, such as a clinical response to hormonal therapy in breast cancers; (2) previously validated methods, such as one of the biochemical assays for estrogen receptor content; or (3) comparison to a valid standard. In the case of histochemical testing, comparison with one of several established biochemical assays would seem to be a necessary first step and these comparisons would, when possible, be complemented by comparison with clinical response to hormonal manipulation. One must clearly set forth the criteria for the positivity of any particular specimen and precisely define the controls used to define saturability and specificity. The stability and purity of reagents must be defined and controlled. There is no reason to accept results which have neglected such controls. All histochemical studies of ligand binding must include an evaluation of: (1) percent of cells with positive staining; (2) intensity of individual cell staining; (3) effects of displacement studies using saturating levels of unlabeled hormone on percent cells staining and on staining intensity; (4) effects of temperature on staining characteristics; and (5) effects of fixation and washing on staining characteristics. Only after these parameters have been evaluated and compared to a defined quantity can one establish appropriate limits for assignment of a histochemical specimen as positive or negative.

Once the experimental data have been collected, calculations to establish the reliability of this information should be performed. Necessary computations are (1) sensitivity [true-positive (TP)/TP + false-negative (FN)]; (2) specificity [true-negative (TN)/TN + false-positive (FP)]; (3) predictive value of a positive (TP/TP + FP); and (4) predictive value of a negative (TN/TN + FN). Additionally, intraobserver reproducibility should be evaluated by reexamining specimens and comparing these results with data obtained on initial review; interobserver reproducibility is checked by separate evaluation of specimens by two or more qualified persons and comparison of results. Conflicting results must be reevaluated by involved parties to verify first impressions.

Reagent stability is a critical component in dealing with these procedures. The fluorescent media must demonstrate an acceptable half-life of emission to provide sufficient time for an adequate evaluation. It is essential to ensure batch-to-batch staining consistency by including standards in each analysis. Staining characteristics of the standard must be consistent with each group of specimens examined.

The importance of utilizing the above or similar methods in testing histochemical procedures cannot be overemphasized. Much of the controversy in the literature today in this area is due to conclusions drawn from studies lacking proper data analyses. For each study, the range of positivity and controls utilized should be carefully delineated and studies in which adequate controls are not defined should be rejected. All physiologic definitions of estrogen receptor must include the concept of saturability. The inability to show saturability indicates that the observed binding is not estrogen receptor. Specificity, sensitivity, and predictive values should be calculated. Selection of standards and ability to trace such standards to a universal standard, a biologic response, or a previously validated test method are critical.

## IV. BIOCHEMICAL EVALUATION OF THE ESTROGEN RECEPTOR

### A. Methods

Various methods have been used to detect the presence of ER protein in both normal and cancerous tissues, including protamine precipitation,[13] gel filtration,[14] gel electrophoresis,[15] dextran-coated charcoal assay, and DEAE absorption assay.[15,16] All of these procedures have achieved some success in providing reproducible data. The technique which has proven most reliable and reproducible and which has become the principal method in use today is the dextran-coated charcoal assay (DCCA).[17] This assay involves a multiconcentration titration binding analysis of $^3$H-estradiol to cytosol homogenate protein extracts followed by removal of free $^3$H-estradiol with dextran-coated charcoal. The demonstration of saturability is an integral part of this analysis with parallel incubations to include saturating levels of unlabeled hormone. The data are analyzed by one of a variety of methods (e.g., Scatchard or Woosley Muldoon plots) to quantitate the number of receptor sites per unit volume of cytosol. This is corrected for nonsaturable binding and expressed as binding per milligram of protein or gram DNA present in the sample. In addition, studies using sucrose density gradient (SDG) sedimentation analyses have further characterized the physical parameters of estrogen receptor protein with useful clinical significance.[9]

## B. Biochemical Characteristics of ER

The generally accepted mechanism of steroid hormone action begins with regulation of serum levels of steroid hormones. Steroid binding proteins present in the blood have various affinities and binding capacities for sex steroids. Levels of these proteins influence the amount of serum steroid and, thus, the amount of steroid available to individual cells. These binding proteins vary widely in their specificity, from the nonspecific high capacity binding observed with albumin and prealbumin to the relative high specificity (but still high capacity) of testosterone-estrogen-binding protein.[18] Binding proteins compose one element influencing relative steroid availability to various tissues or organs.

Although it has been suggested that facilitated transport of steroid hormone mediated by plasma membrane receptors occurs, most evidence points toward passive diffusion of steroid across the cytoplasmic membrane once the hormone reaches the cell. Upon entering the cytoplasm, the steroid molecule may bind to one of several proteins which are capable of binding sex steroids.[15,17] Binding to the "classical" estrogen receptor (ER) causes activation of the receptor by mechanisms which have not been elucidated.[19-23] These activated molecules show a strong tendency to concentrate in the nuclear compartment. In the nucleus, the activated steroid-receptor complex binds to "nuclear acceptor", a term embracing the many sites with which this complex has been observed to bind.[24-28] This variation in location of nuclear binding has led to the suggestion that differences in tissues may exist at the level of nuclear interaction. This issue is at present poorly understood, as are the mechanisms by which chromatin binding influences transcriptional control. The particular effect nuclear binding of receptor-steroid complex will have on a cell depends on the steroid, the type of cell, and the physiologic state of the host (e.g., circulating level of hormone, duration of exposure).

As a result of various studies, receptor binding proteins have generally been divided into three classes, largely based on relative capacity and affinity. Type I binding, the "classical" estrogen receptor protein, is present only in estrogen-responsive cells and is characterized by a sedimentation coefficient of 8S in low salt sucrose density gradients.[15,17] Activated ER involves a temperature-dependent transformation and translocation from the cytoplasm to the nucleus influencing transcription.[29] Type I receptor has been shown to bind estrogen in a stereospecific manner with high affinity ($K_d$'s = $10^{-11}$ to $10^{-9}$ $M$) and limited capacity.[30] The sedimentation coefficient in low salt gradients for this nuclear form of the receptor is in the 5S range.[31] The number of receptor sites varies from 1,000 to 20,000 per cell.[15] An important criterion for recognizing the steroid specificity of $^3$H-estradiol in binding to these receptors is the ability to show defined capacity of binding by unlabeled estradiol or estrogen analogs (saturability), while specificity is demonstrated by the absence of inhibition even by high concentrations of other classes of steroid hormones.[32] Type II binding demonstrates a lower affinity as well as a higher capacity than type I binding and is usually manifested at ligand concentrations of $10^{-8}$ to $10^{-7}$ $M$.[33] These proteins appear to have sedimentation coefficients of 4 to 5S in low salt SDG. Estradiol concentrations in the range of $10^{-7}$ $M$ are required to saturate these sites because of their high capacity. Additional ubiquitous, nonspecific binding sites within cells such as prealbumin, sex-hormone binding globulin, and membrane-associated molecules are associated with type III binding sites.[30] The binding capacities of these can exceed steroid solubility in aqueous media which necessitate ligand concentrations of $10^{-7}$ to $10^{-5}$ $M$ for binding. There is no evidence that type III sites are involved in translocation or transcription. Any studies which necessitate micromolar concentrations of steroid are unlikely to be directly involved in the regulation of transcription.

## C. Limitations

In discussing the analysis of ER it is important to note certain procedural limitations. For example, the SDG analysis is costly in terms of equipment and technician time. These factors may preclude use of this method in all but larger medical centers. The titration analyses require a minimum of 100 mg of wet tissue, an amount which may be difficult to obtain with effusion cells or needle aspirates.

For a number of reasons, false-negative results may occur in both the DCCA and SDG procedures. Some errors may result from procedural mishaps or misinterpretation of methodology.[34] Improper storage and handling of the specimens may result in a decrease in observed binding due to thermolability. Inherent in the technical procedure for the biochemical assay is an inability to determine the source or proportion of cells from a heterogenous cell population which is demonstrating binding activity. Some authors have justifiably raised the issue of variability of receptor content from histologically comparable areas of the same tumor.[35] Dissociation of estrogen receptor and ligand during ultracentrifugation is another possible source of lowered quantitation.[34] Finally, it has been noted that biopsies from different sites in a single patient may yield varying results.

"Biologic false-positives" also constitute a point of concern with the present analyses. These cases occur when ER-positive tumors are unresponsive to hormonal therapy. Several factors may play a role in these phenomena. Breast tumors have been suggested to be heterogenous, composed of both endocrine-dependent and endocrine-independent cells.[36] In theory, a tumor containing few highly ER-positive cells could give a positive assay result, while the physiologic response and hormone therapy would be dictated by the majority of ER-negative cells.[34] In addition, it should be remembered that principally cytoplasmic receptor is measured by the biochemical assays, while the manifestation of hormonal response occurs via a complex pathway in which cytoplasmic receptor plays only one part. Factors which interfere with the cytoplasm to nuclear translocation mechanism after steroid-receptor binding, such as inhibitory factors or defective nuclear acceptors, have been suggested as possible points of pathway interference.[34,37] Accordingly, postreceptor-binding markers have been sought to augment ER analyses.[24,37-39] Additional factors which may induce false positive results include the effect of nonsteroid hormones on tumor response,[40] the tendency for metastases to exhibit decreased receptor content over time in relation to the primary lesion, host tumor relationships important in influencing remission, and failure to strictly observe criteria for determining objective remissions.

Despite the above problems, the DCCA and SDG analyses clearly represent the most well-documented and effective procedures for ER determination because of their reproducibility and reliability. Although variability has been shown to exist among laboratories in reporting ER values,[41] especially in borderline cases, quality control mechanisms such as interlaboratory comparisons and cytosol standards make these two assays the procedures of choice.[42,43]

An interesting point in considering variability of ER status among different patients with similar tumors is the menopausal status. The high degree of ER negativity in premenopausal patients has been attributed by some to high levels of endogenous estrogens occupying receptor sites. The expected result of surgical oophorectomy or natural menopause would, thus, be conversion to ER-positive status. However, in paramenopausal women (1 to 4 years after the last menstrual period) developing breast tumors, the absence of ER positivity has been shown to be below that of either pre- or postmenopausal women.[44] Furthermore, the expected conversion to ER-positive status after menopause has not been observed, indicating that factors other than endogenous estrogens operate in paramenopausal lesions. This is entirely compatible with clinical observations concerning the relatively lower hormonal response frequency of paramenopausal women who develop breast tumors. Physiologic status of the patient must be considered when evaluating possible reasons for resistance of ER-positive tumors to hormonal manipulation.

### D. Clinical Correlations

With the advent of estrogen receptor assays as a predictor of clinical response to hormonal therapy, the objective remission rate for hormonal therapies has risen from 20 to 30% using clinical criteria alone and to 55 to 60% using only estrogen receptor as a marker.[17,45] Subsequently, further clinical testing has shown the presence of estrogen receptor to correlate with better differentiated tumors,[46,47] longer disease-free intervals,[48] and better survival rates.[49,50] Estrogen-receptor negative tumors have proven to be more anaplastic, more likely to recur, and show shorter survival rates than ER-positive lesions.[11,49,51] Several investigators have shown that ER-negative tumors seem to be more likely to be associated with visceral metastases than ER-positive tumors.[11,51] There has been speculation that ER-negative tumors could prove more susceptible to chemotherapy than ER-positive tumors.[52] Reasoning for this argument stems from data showing that tumors with rapid cellular proliferation are usually ER negative, combined with the knowledge that rapidly proliferating tumors are usually fairly responsive to chemotherapy. Whether the conclusions drawn from this information are valid remains controversial.[53-55]

As mentioned above, postreceptor-binding markers are proving to be clinically useful as a supplement to ER determinations. Patients whose breast tumors contain significant amounts of both estrogen and progesterone receptors have a response rate of nearly 90% to sex steroid manipulation.[39,56]

## V. HISTOLOGIC CORRELATIONS WITH ER

Correlation of various histologic parameters of human breast tumors with status of estrogen receptor assay has been a much studied area, although few consistently observed relationships have emerged.

### A. Tumor Type

Several studies have indicated a trend towards a greater incidence of positive ER assays in invasive lobular carcinomas vs. ductal carcinomas,[57-67] although one recent and comprehensive study shows a much lower incidence.[68] The paucity of cells in classic invasive lobular carcinomas raises questions about the accuracy of assay data, questioning whether relative tumor cellularity is the source of observed differences.

Colloid carcinoma studies have also produced conflicting reports. While four studies,[46,57,58,68] including two large series, have reported an incidence of ER positivity in colloid carcinomas of 33 to 56%, six other reports have found consistent ER positivity in these lesions.[59,61-64,66]

Medullary carcinomas have shown a uniformly low incidence of ER positivity, with all reported incidences being well below 50% with the exception of Nishimura et al. (56% positive).[66] It has been suggested that this may bear some relationship to the high incidence of lymphocytic stromal invasion characteristic of these tumors.[69]

The rare tubular carcinoma has been studied only in small numbers, and results of these studies range from consistent negative findings to consistently positive results.[58,63]

Studies of other receptors in breast carcinomas have lagged behind those of estrogen receptor. Three series addressing progesterone receptor (PR) content of various breast tumors have shown only a slight trend toward PR negativity in medullary and colloid carcinomas.[46,62,66]

## B. Tumor Grade

Although the number of grading systems used by authors studying correlation of histologic and nuclear tumor grades with ER status makes comparisons difficult, a definite trend towards a higher incidence of ER positivity in well-differentiated carcinomas as compared to poorly differentiated tumors exists.[57,58,60,62,63,66-68,70-74]

Many reports indicate that nuclear grading relates more closely to the presence of sex steroid receptor than does any other single histologic factor.[46,75,76] Well-differentiated tumors, as evaluated by nuclear grade, have a significantly higher incidence of ER positivity than do poorly differentiated lesions. An interesting cytological correlate to the usefulness of histologic nuclear grading in predicting ER status is the calculation of mean nuclear areas in thin-needle aspirates from breast carcinomas. Measuring the nuclear diameters of cells obtained by thin-needle aspirations from a series of breast tumors, while evaluating the histologic grade of excisional biopsies removed concurrently, revealed that mean nuclear area calculations correlated more closely with ER positivity than did histologic grade.[76]

Progesterone receptors have also proved to correlate with histologic grading. Several groups have shown a positive correlation between incidence of PR positivity and better differentiated tumors.[62,77] In contrast to ER studies, no predictable trends have yet been identified comparing nuclear grade and PR status.[78]

The availability of well-documented specific biochemical assays for steroid receptors diminishes the importance of trying to predict receptor content utilizing histologic parameters of questionable predictive value. Correlations with such histologic parameters, however, should continue to prove useful in establishing response or prognostic trends in ER-containing lesions of different histologic grades as well as in furthering our comprehension of the biology of human breast cancers.

## C. Other Histologic Features

Ductal carcinomas frequently exhibit elastosis around involved ducts, termed periductal elastosis.[79] This entity has been shown by several investigators to correlate positively with ER content;[62,67,73,80-82] however, a recent well-structured study by Reyes et al.[83] did not demonstrate any appreciable correlation with ER status.

Infiltration of tumor stroma by lymphocytes has been claimed to be prognostically important.[84] Evidence has accumulated to suggest that this stromal invasion may be inversely correlated with ER positivity in some tumors.[57,58,62,63,65,66,68,73] The scirrhous variant of infiltrating ductal carcinoma is known to be consistently negative for ER when lymphocytic infiltration occurred in these tumors. The observation that medullary carcinomas frequently fail to demonstrate estrogen receptors may be the consequence of the fact that these tumors characteristically show dense stromal lymphocytic invasion.[69] No consistent relationships between other forms of carcinoma and stromal infiltrates have been detected.

The relative cellularity of various tumors has proved troublesome in interpreting biochemical assays for ER. The expectation that ER positivity would increase with increasing tumor cellularity has not been fulfilled; two studies showed a lower incidence of ER positivity in highly cellular tumors than in low cellularity lesions.[63,80] However, the trend shown by many of the published studies correlates ER positivity with increasing cellularity.[57,58,60,67,70] These observations emphasize the desirability of developing an acceptable histochemical assay.

## VI. HISTOLOGIC CORRELATION WITH OTHER SUBSTANCES

The search for additional biochemical correlates of histologic differentiation to supplement ER and PR analysis has led to examination of several different substances for this purpose. Two such proteins, the gross cystic disease fluid protein (GCDFP-15) and the nonreceptor progesterone-binding protein (PBP), were compared with ER and PR in a correlation with degree of tumor differentiation.[85] Both of these substances parallel the trend demonstrated by sex steroid receptor to decrease in less well-differentiated tumors.

## VII. HISTOCHEMISTRY

### A. Considerations

As a preface to discussing the applications of histochemical staining for receptor proteins, the minimum criteria of any histochemical assay for estrogen receptor must be considered. A ligand (steroid or steroid analog) proposed for use in steroid receptor assay, histochemical or otherwise, should be evaluated to determine several parameters. These include proper competition studies to demonstrate the binding affinity and ligand specificity.

Firm evidence of specific binding interaction must be demonstrated, with binding confined to target tissues. Identification by sedimentation coefficient may contribute to characterization of the binding species interacting with the ligand in question.[15,17] The evaluation of titration data from binding of receptor of labeled steroid derivative should show high affinity with finite capacity (i.e., a definite saturation point). This finite number of binding sites is a fundamental characteristic of receptor proteins. It is essential that there should be acceptable agreement with established assays and/or correlation with observed clinical response.

A consideration which is always important in histochemical procedures is the type of specimen chosen and the method of fixation for that tissue. Because of the known thermolability of estrogen receptor, many investigators have used unfixed frozen sections for their procedures.[36,86-95] In view of the aqueous solubility of steroid receptor and other cytoplasmic constituents, the validity of using cells whose cytoplasmic and nuclear membranes have been disrupted through freezing in a procedure involving incubation with various aqueous solutions must be questioned. A study by Lee[96] designed to address this problem claimed to show that ER does, indeed, remain in frozen sections incubated with an aqueous mediacontaining $^3$H-estradiol at 4°C. However, some of the data from these experiments bear close scrutiny. As pointed out by Underwood,[69] estradiol binding claiming to be specific continued to rise for up to 48 hr during testing, a finding at odds with the tendency of soluble receptor proteins to diffuse into an aqueous solution after the cell membrane is made permeable by freezing or sectioning. Therefore, in light of present knowledge, histochemical "receptor-localizing" procedures involving unfixed, cryostat-sectioned tissues must be interpreted with caution.

Frozen sections as well as permanent sections treated with various fixatives have also been used in these investigations. In a study by Raam et al.,[97] acetone, formaldehyde, Bouin's solution, and 95% ethanol were all shown to significantly reduce the specific binding capacity of ER in frozen sections. Only graded alcohols preserved the receptor adequately for apparent localization. Other investigations lend credence to these observations.[98,99] Preincubation of frozen sections with estradiol prior to formalin fixation has been suggested to protect ER from alteration.[100] It was proposed that the bound estradiol would then be solubilized from the receptor by the solvents used in paraffin embedding. The quantitative accuracy of procedures using various methods of fixation must be tested for each ligand and/or antibody used.

It is important to note that some problems relating to the biochemical assay also extend to histochemical procedures, in particular, the concept of tumor heterogeneity. If histologically similar areas of the same tumors yield varying biochemical receptor assay results, it is reasonable to assume that sections or cells from different areas of a tumor may show different histochemical characteristics. A method to compensate for potential errors in this regard, and a means to quantify such "error" such as staining of sections from several areas of the tumor in question, would be necessary should an acceptable histochemical procedure be developed.

## B. Methods

### 1. Ligand-Antibody Method

Several investigators have used immunocytochemical methods with antibody directed against the sex steroid in attempts to localize ER on frozen sections or in fresh tumor cells.[24,36,37,86,88,89,91,93,100-107] Tissues are initially incubated with estradiol or estrogen derivatives, followed by washing and incubation with antiestradiol antibodies. Either this antibody or a second antibody "tagged" with a fluorescein- or peroxidase-linked secondary antibody is used for visualization. The use of frozen sections brings into play previous criticisms concerning diffusion and/or extraction of estrogen receptor in aqueous media, although several studies have used fixed tissues. The question of the availability of receptor-bound estradiol to antiestradiol antibodies must also be raised. Evidence suggests the reaction between estrogen receptor and estradiol is clathrate; that is, the estradiol is "enveloped" by receptor in a process which involves a conformational change of receptor. Several investigations, including a convincing study by Morrow et al.,[108] indicate that this altered estradiol-receptor complex is not capable of reacting with antiestradiol antibodies in vivo or in vitro.[109,110] Attempts to maximize the antigenic surface of the steroid by use of polymerized polyestradiol phosphate (PEP) by Pertschuk have been met with much criticism and have been discontinued.[105,110-112] It seems likely that steroid bound to nonspecific type II or type III receptors is more accessible to antibody than is estradiol bound to ER. It follows that any staining procedure utilizing antiestradiol antibodies would be more likely to detect nonspecific binding than ER-bound estradiol.

Another criticism of these methods must be directed at the concentrations of estradiol and inhibitors used.[30] Competitive inhibition studies are an important component for demonstrating the specificity of a ligand for ER. Many laboratories have reported inhibition of staining using DES or antiestrogens;[88,89] however, in each case, the high concentrations of inhibitors used makes likely the replacement of labeled type II and type III binding in addition to inhibition of any labeled ER-bound ligand. Even at these concentrations, inhibition could not be considered complete. Primary ligand concentrations used by many laboratories in these studies have also been extraordinarily high.[30] It is well established that saturation of estrogen receptors occurs at estradiol concentrations of approximately $10^{-9} M$. At higher concentrations, the only additional receptors bound are the low-affinity, high-capacity type II (above $10^{-9} M$) and type III (above $10^{-7} M$) varieties.[33] Despite this knowledge, high concentrations of estradiol ($10^{-4}$ to $10^{-8} M$) have been used in several studies, making likely the occurrence of nonspecific binding.[100,101,105,106] One study which did use an estradiol concentration of $10^{-9} M$ showed no fluorescence by histochemical means.[113] Realistic concentrations of both ligand ($10^{-9} M$) and inhibitor ($10^{-8}$ to $10^{-7} M$) must be maintained in order to obtain useful information from histochemical studies of ER binding.

Two studies claiming correlation of ligand-antibody histochemical methods with accepted biochemical assays have been reported.[105,114] Using the data from these reports, the calculation of sensitivities and specificities compared with SDG analyses shows unacceptably low values for the specificity of these procedures (Table 1).[115]

Demonstrations of temperature-dependent translocation of labeled ER complex from cytoplasm to nucleus using immunocytochemical methods have been reported,[24,37,101] while others have failed to corroborate these findings.[116] Increased nuclear localization noted in these tests has been arbitrarily attributed to an increase in nuclear type II "receptor" after estrogen treatment, a concept without scientific proof as there is no evidence of translocation of type II binding.[30] An important study by Mercer et al.[113] failed to show a reduction in cytoplasmic immunofluorescence after treating human breast cancer cells with DES, despite having shown biochemical evidence that true ER had been translocated to the nucleus. This indicates that the method used was most likely detecting some nonspecific binding.

**Table 1**
## COMPARISON OF HISTOCHEMICAL TO
## SUCROSE GRADIENT RECEPTOR ANALYSES

|  | Sensitivity[a] | Specificity[a] |
|---|---|---|
| Poly-E$_2$/anti-E$_2$ | 53.5 | 45.4 |
| 6 BSA-fluor-CMO-17β-estradiol | 60.0 | 57.6 |
| 17 BSA-fluor-HS-estrogen | 86.7 | 48.5 |

[a] Calculations based on comparisons of histochemical technique to standard gradient technique.[116] Sensitivity = 100 × true-pos/(true-pos + false-neg); specificity = 100 × true-neg/(true-neg + false-pos). For abbreviations, see Table 2 legend.

No relation between immunocytochemical staining using antisteroid antibody to demonstrate estrogen binding and clinical response to hormonal therapy has been adequately established.

### 2. Labeled Ligand Method

Efforts to circumvent the questionable binding of antiestrogen antibody to the receptor-estradiol complex have led some workers to directly label estradiol with fluorescein substances or to use a substituted estradiol compound linked to fluoresceinated albumin molecules. Some of the compounds involved include estradiol linked directly to fluorescein via a 6-carboxymethyloxime or 17-β-hemisuccinate bridge, and similar 6-CMO and 17-β-HS bridges linking estradiol to a fluorescein-BSA substance.[87,89,117]

Some of the same criticisms of ligand-antibody methods are applicable to labeled ligand testing. Data are lacking to demonstrate use of an appropriate K$_d$, performance of appropriate competition experiments using reasonable concentrations of ligand and competitors, and binding to an 8S species on SDG analysis for these fluoresceinated compounds. Specifically, the relative calculated binding affinities of the various compounds used are unacceptably low (Table 2).[111,118,119] Ligand concentrations used in the reports of the histochemical ER localization studies were 100 to 1000 times as great as the calculated K$_d$s, again suggesting nonspecific binding. Competitive inhibition of the fluorescein-BSA-linked estradiol compound was achieved by Pertschuk[89,104] by using $10^3$ to $10^4$ as much as the reported K$_d$s. The problem of how a ligand molecule with one to five fluorescein molecules per receptor molecule (1000 to 20,000 receptor sites per cell) can be visualized has not been resolved.[15]

Basic procedural problems must again be raised in reference to these methods. Diffusion of soluble receptor proteins from damaged cells into aqueous incubation media remains of concern. The ability of specific receptor site to identify and bind with ligand which has been altered by the addition of a large radical group is questionable. A study by Penney and Hawkins of labeled albumin-estradiol conjugates showed no specificity and a low binding affinity for these compounds.[98]

Of possible promise are studies by Pertschuk et al.[36] utilizing coumestrol, a naturally fluorescent plant estrogen, effective against breast and prostatic tumors. Using appropriate concentrations, a weak fluorescence which was apparently repressed by nonfluorescent estradiol but not by other steroid hormones was observed.

### C. Receptor-Antibody Methods

Perhaps the most promise in the field of histochemical detection of estrogen receptors lies in the use of monoclonal antibodies against estrogen receptor. The availability of such reagents opens a whole new horizon for receptor localization with well-characterized methods for amplification to allow visualization of antibody localized on tissue sections. With these

## Table 2
## RELATIVE BINDING AFFINITIES OF FLUORESCENT
## LABELED LIGANDS

| Compound | Relative affinity[a] |
|---|---|
| 17β-Estradiol | 1.000 |
| 17 Fluor-ethyl-HS-estrogen | 0.150[b] |
| 17 Fluor-TSC-estrogen | 0.030[c] |
| 17 BSA-fluor-HS-estrogen | 0.015 |
| 17 BSA-HS-estrogen | 0.015 |
| 17 BSA-fluor-butryl-estrogen | <0.001 |
| 6 BSA-fluor-CMO-17β-estradiol | <0.001 |
| 6 Fluor-CMO-17β-estradiol | <0.003[c] |
| Polyestradiol phosphate | <0.001 |
| (After partial hydrolysis) | 0.01 |

[a] Ratio of the molar concentration of 17β-estradiol to compound required to reduce estradiol binding to half its initial value.[116] Fluor = fluorescein isothiocyanate; HS = hemisuccinate; TSC = thiosemicarbazone; BSA = bovine serum albumin; CMO = carboxymethyloxime.

[b] As reported by Barrows et al.[118]

[c] As reported by Dandliker et al.[119]

techniques, the binding of antibody does not require the preservation of the thermolabile steroid binding site of the receptor protein. The results of such anti-$E_2$ receptor antibody localization experiments are an area warranting close scrutiny because of their great promise to further our understanding of the biology of sex steroid action in health and disease.

## REFERENCES

1. **Jensen, E. V. and Jacobson, H. I.,** Fate of steroid receptors in target tissue, in *Biologic Activity of Steroids in Relation to Cancer,* Pincus, G., and Vollmer, E. B., Eds., Academic Press, New York, 1960, 161.
2. **Folca, P. J., Glascock, R. F., and Irving, W. T.,** Studies with tritium-labelled hexoestrol in advanced breast cancer, *Lancet,* 2, 796, 1961.
3. **Toft, D. and Gorski, J.,** A receptor molecule for estrogens: isolation from the rat uterus and preliminary characterization, *Proc. Natl. Acad. Sci. U.S.A.,* 55, 1574, 1966.
4. **Beatson, G. T.,** On the treatment of inoperable cases of the mammae: suggestions for alternative method of treatment with illustrative cases, *Lancet,* 2, 104, 1896.
5. **Huggins, C. and Bergenstal, D. M.,** Inhibition of human mammary and prostatic cancer by adrenalectomy, *Cancer Res.,* 12, 134, 1952.
6. **Luft, R. and Olivecrona, H.,** Hypophysectomy in man: experience in metastatic cancer of the breast, *Cancer,* 8, 261, 1955.
7. **Jensen, E. V., De Sombre, E. R., and Jungblut, P. W. P.,** *Estrogen in Hormone Responsive Tissue and Tumors,* University of Chicago Press, Illinois, 1967.
8. **Dao, T. L. and Nemoto, T.,** Steroid receptors and response to endocrine ablations in women with metastatic cancer of the breast, *Cancer,* 46, 2779, 1980.
9. **McCarty, K. S., Jr., Cox, C., Silva, J. S. et al.,** Comparison of sex steroid receptor analysis and carcinoembryonic antigen with clinical response to hormone therapy, *Cancer,* 46, 2847, 1980.
10. **Rubens, R. D. and Hayward, J. L.,** Estrogen receptors and response to endocrine therapy and cytotoxic chemotherapy in advanced breast cancer, *Cancer,* 46, 2922, 1980.
11. **Singhakowinta, A., Saunders, D. E., Brooks, S. C. et al.,** Clinical applications of estrogen receptor in breast cancer, *Cancer,* 46, 2932, 1980.
12. **Galen, R. S. and Gambino, S. R.,** *Beyond Normality: The Predictive Value and Efficiency of Medical Diagnosis,* John Wiley & Sons, New York, 1975.

13. **Lippman, M. E. and Huff, K.,** A demonstration of androgen and estrogen receptor using a new protamine sulfate assay, *Cancer,* 38, 868, 1976.

14. **Godefroi, V. C. and Brooks, S. C.,** Improved gel filtration method for analysis of estrogen binding, *Ann. Biochem.,* 51, 335, 1973.

15. **McCarty, K. S., Jr. and McCarty, K. S., Sr.,** Steroid hormone receptors in the regulation of differentiation, *Am. J. Pathol.,* 86, 705, 1977.

16. **McGuire, W. L.,** Estrogen receptor in human breast cancer, *J. Clin. Invest.,* 52, 73, 1973.

17. **McGuire, W. L., Vollmer, E. P., and Carbone, P. P., Eds.,** *Estrogen Receptors in Human Breast Cancer,* Raven Press, New York, 1975.

18. **Westphal, U.,** Steroid-protein interactions, in *Monographs on Endocrinology,* Vol. 4, Springer-Verlag, New York, 1971.

19. **Shyamala, G. and Gorski, J.,** Estrogen receptors in the rat uterus: studies on the interaction of cytosol and nuclear binding sites, *J. Biol. Chem.,* 244, 1097, 1969.

20. **Lukola, A., Punnonen, R., and Tahtinen, U.,** Salt-induced transformation of the human myometrial estrogen receptor, *J. Steroid Biochem.,* 4, 1241, 1981.

21. **Milgrom, E.,** Activation of steroid-receptor complexes, in *Biochemical Actions of Steroid Hormones,* Litkin, G., Ed., Academic Press, New York, 1981, 465.

22. **Auricchio, F., Migliaccio, A., and Potondi, A.,** Inactivation of oestrogen receptor in vitro by nuclear dephosphorylation, *Biochem. J.,* 194, 569, 1981.

23. **Weigel, N. L., Schrader, W. T., and O'Malley, B. W.,** Progesterone receptor: functional domains and phosphorylation, in *Programme and Abstract of 64th Annual Endocrine Society Meeting,* 1982.

24. **Nenci, I.,** Receptor and nucleolar pathways of steroid action in normal and neoplastic cells, *Cancer Res.,* 38, 4204, 1978.

25. **Scott, R. W. and Frankel, F. R.,** Enrichment of estradiol-receptor complexes in a transcriptionally active fraction of chromatin from MCF-7 cells, *Proc. Natl. Acad. Sci. U.S.A.,* 77, 1291, 1980.

26. **Kallos, J., Fasy, T. M., and Hollander, V. P.,** Assessment of estrogen receptor-histone interactions, *Proc. Natl. Acad. Sci. U.S.A.,* 78, 2874, 1981.

27. **Barrack, E. R. and Coffey, D. S.,** Biological properties of the nuclear matrix: steroid hormone binding, *Recent Prog. Horm. Res.,* 38, 133, 1982.

28. **Compton, J. G., Schrader, W. T., and O'Malley, B. W.,** Selective binding of chicken progesterone receptor A subunit to a DNA fragment containing ovalbumin gene sequences, *Biochem. Biophys. Res. Comm.,* 105, 96, 1982.

29. **Markaverich, B. M. and Clark, J. H.,** Quantitation of nuclear estrogen receptors in the rat uterus by ($^3$H)-estradiol exchange, *J. Steroid Biochem.,* 15, 289, 1981.

30. **Chamness, G. C., Mercer, W. D., and McGuire, W. L.,** Are histochemical methods for estrogen receptor valid?, *J. Histochem. Cytochem.,* 28, 792, 1980.

31. **Gorski, J., Toft, D., Shyamala, G. et al.,** Hormone receptors: studies on the interaction of estrogen with the uterus, *Recent Prog. Horm. Res.,* 24, 45, 1968.

32. **McGuire, W. L. and Julian, J. A.,** Comparison of macromolecular binding of estradiol in hormone-dependent and hormone independent rat mammary carcinoma, *Cancer Res.,* 31, 1440, 1971.

33. **Clark, J. H., Hardin, J. W., Upchurch, S., and Eriksson, H.,** Heterogeneity of estrogen binding sites in the cytosol of the rat uterus, *J. Biol. Chem.,* 253, 7630, 1978.

34. **Lippman, M. E. and Allegra, J. C.,** Receptors in breast cancer, *N. Engl. J. Med.,* 299, 930, 1978.

35. **Poulsen, H. S.,** Oestrogen receptor assay — limitation of method, *Eur. J. Cancer,* 17, 495, 1981.

36. **Pertschuk, L. P., Tobin, E. H., Tanapat, P., et al.,** Histochemical analysis of steroid hormone receptors in breast and prostatic carcinoma, *J. Histochem. Cytochem.,* 28, 799, 1980.

37. **Nenci, I., Beccati, M. D., and Pagnini, C. A.,** Estrogen receptors and post receptor markers in human breast cancer: a reappraisal, *Tumori,* 64, 161, 1978.

38. **McGuire, W. L., Horwitz, K. B., Pearson, O. H., and Segaloff, A.,** Current status of estrogen and progesterone receptors in breast cancer, *Cancer,* 39, 2934, 1977.

39. **Young, P. C. M., Ehrlich, C. E., Einhorn, L. H.,** Relationship between steroid receptors and response to endocrine therapy and cytotoxic chemotherapy in metastatic breast cancer, *Cancer,* 46, 2961, 1980.

40. **Costlow, M. E., Buschow, R. A., and McGuire, W. L.,** Prolactin receptors in an estrogen receptor-deficient mammary carcinoma, *Science,* 184, 85, 1974.

41. **King, R. J. B.,** Quality control of estradiol receptor analysis: the United Kingdom experience, *Cancer,* 46, 2822, 1980.

42. **Bojar, H., Staib, W., Beck, K., and Pelaski, J.,** Investigation on the thermostability of steroid hormone receptors in lyophilized calf uterine powders, *Cancer,* 46, 2270, 1980.

43. **Smith, R. G.,** Quality control in steroid hormone receptor assays, *Cancer,* 46, 2946, 1980.

44. **Kiang, D. T., and Kennedy, B. J.,** Factors affecting estrogen receptors in breast cancer, *Cancer,* 40, 1571, 1977.

45. **Harris, H. S. and Spratt, J. S.,** Bilateral adrenalectomy in metastatic mammary cancer, *Cancer,* 23, 145, 1969.
46. **McCarty, K. S., Jr., Barton, T. K., Fetter, B. F., et al.,** Correlation of estrogen and progesterone receptors with histologic differentiation in mammary carcinoma, *Cancer,* 46, 2851, 1980.
47. **Maynard, P. V., Davies, C. J., Blamey, R. W., et al.,** Relationship between oestrogen-receptor content and histologic grade in human primary breast tumors, *Br. J. Cancer,* 38, 745, 1978.
48. **Knight, W. A., Livingston, R. B., Gregory, E. J., and McGuire, W. L.,** Estrogen receptor as an independent prognostic factor for early recurrence in breast cancer, *Cancer Res.,* 37, 4669, 1977.
49. **Furmanski, P., Saunders, D. E., Brooks, S. C., et al.,** The prognostic value of estrogen receptor in patients with primary breast cancer, *Cancer,* 46, 2794, 1980.
50. **Blamey, R. W., Bishops, H. M., Blake, J. R. S., et al.,** Relationships between primary tumor receptor status and patient survival, *Cancer,* 46, 2765, 1980.
51. **Walt, A. J., Singhakowinta, A., Brooks, S. C., and Cortez, A.,** The surgical implications of estrophile protein estimations in carcinoma of the breast, *Surgery,* 80, 506, 1976.
52. **Meyer, J. S., Rao, B. R., Stevens, S. C., and White, W. L.,** Low incidence of estrogen receptor in breast carcinoma with rapid rates of cellular replication, *Cancer,* 40, 2209, 1977.
53. **Rosenbaum, C., Marsland, T. A., Stolbach, L. L. et al.,** Estrogen receptor status and response to chemotherapy in advanced breast cancer, *Cancer,* 46, 2919, 1980.
54. **Rubens, R. D. and Hayward, J. L.,** Estrogen receptors and response to endocrine therapy and cytotoxic chemotherapy in advanced breast cancer, *Cancer,* 46, 2922, 1980.
55. **Samal, B. A., Brooks, S. C., Cummings, G. et al.,** Estrogen receptors and responsiveness of advanced breast cancer to chemotherapy, *Cancer,* 46, 2925, 1980.
56. **Skinner, L. G., Barnes, D. M., and Ribeiro, G. G.,** The clinical value of multiple steroid receptor assays in breast cancer management, *Cancer,* 46, 2939, 1980.
57. **Rosen, P. P., Mendez-Botet, C. J., Nisselbaum, J. S. et al.,** Pathological review of breast lesions analysed for estrogen receptor protein, *Cancer Res.,* 35, 3187, 1975.
58. **Rosen, P. P., Mendez-Botet, C. J., Senie, R. T. et al.,** Estrogen receptor protein (ERP) and the histo-pathology of human mammary carcinoma, in *Hormones, Receptors, and Breast Cancer,* McGuire, W. L., Ed., Raven Press, New York, 1978, 71.
59. **Meyer, J. S., Bauer, W. C., and Rao, B. R.,** Subpopulations of breast carcinoma defined by S-phase fraction, morphology and estrogen receptor content, *Lab. Invest.,* 39, 225, 1978.
60. **Antoniades, K. and Spector, H.,** Correlation of estrogen receptor levels with histology and cytomorphology in human mammary cancer, *Am. J. Clin. Pathol.,* 71, 497, 1979.
61. **Kern, W. H.,** Morphologic and clinical aspects of estrogen receptors in carcinoma of the breast, *Surg. Gynecol. Obstet.,* 148, 240, 1979.
62. **Millis, R. R.,** Correlation of hormone receptors with pathological features in human breast cancer, *Cancer,* 46, 2869, 1980.
63. **Parl, F. F. and Wagner, R. K.,** The histopathological evaluation of human breast cancer in correlation with estrogen receptor values, *Cancer,* 46, 362, 1980.
64. **Silfversward, C., Gustafsson, J.-A., Gustafsson, S. A., et al.,** Estrogen receptor concentrations in 269 cases of histologically classified human breast cancer, *Cancer,* 45, 2001, 1980.
65. **Fu, Y. S., Maksem, J. A., Hubay, C. A. et al.,** The relationship of breast cancer morphology and oestrogen receptor protein status, *Prog. Surg. Pathol.,* 3, 65, 1981.
66. **Nishimura, R., Misumi, A., Kimura, M. et al.,** Relationship between the content of estrogen and progesterone receptors and the pathological characteristics of human breast cancer, *Jpn. J. Surg.,* 12, 191, 1982.
67. **Rasmussen, B. B., Rose, C., Thorpe, S. M. et al.,** Histopathological characteristics of oestrogen receptor content in primary breast carcinoma, *Virchow Arch. (Pathol. Anat. Histol.),* 390, 347, 1981.
68. **Lesser, M. L., Rosen, P. P., Senie, R. T., et ai.,** Estrogen and progesterone receptors in breast carcinoma: correlations with epidemiology and pathology, *Cancer,* 48, 299, 1981.
69. **Underwood, J. C. E.,** Oestrogen receptors in human breast cancer: review of histopathological correlations and critique of histochemical methods, *Diagn. Histopathol.,* 6, 1, 1983.
70. **Terenius, L., Johansson, H., Rimsten, A., and Thoren, L.,** Malignant and benign human mammary disease: estrogen binding in relation to clinical data, *Cancer,* 33, 1363, 1974.
71. **Elston, C. W., Blamey, R. W., Johnson, J. et al.,** The relationship of oestradiol receptor (ER) and histological tumor differentiation with prognosis in human primary breast cancer, *Eur. J. Cancer,* Suppl. 1, 59, 1980.
72. **Thoresen, S., Tangen, M., Stoa, K. F., and Hartveit, F.,** Estrogen receptor values and histological grade in human breast cancer, *Histopathology,* 5, 257, 1981.
73. **Fisher, E. R., Osborne, C. K., McGuire, W. L. et al.,** Correlation of primary breast cancer histopathology and estrogen receptor content, *Br. Cancer Res. Treat.,* 1, 37, 1981.

74. **Mohla, S., Sampson, C. C., Khan, T. et al.,** Estrogen and progesterone receptors in breast cancer in black Americans: correlation of receptor data with tumor differentiation, *Cancer,* 50, 552, 1982.

75. **Mossler, J. A., McCarty, K. S., Jr., and Johnston, W. W.,** The correlation of cytologic grade and steroid receptor content in effusions of metastatic breast cancer, *Acta Cytol.,* 25, 653, 1981.

76. **Mossler, J. A., McCarty, K. S., Jr., Woodard, B. H. et al.,** Correlation of mean nuclear area with estrogen receptor content in aspiration cytology of breast carcinoma, *Acta Cytol.,* 26, 417, 1982.

77. **Martin, P. M., Rolland, P. H., Jacquemier, J. et al.,** Multiple steroid receptor in human breast cancer. III. Relationships between steroid receptors and the state of differentiation and the activities of carcinomas throughout the pathologic features, *Cancer Chemother. Pharmacol.,* 2, 115, 1979.

78. **Syrjanen, K. J. and Kosma, V.-M.,** Hormone receptor levels related to histological parameters of tumour-host relationships in female breast carcinoma, *J. Surg. Oncol.,* 21, 49, 1982.

79. **Azzopardi, J. G., and Laurini, R. N.,** Elastosis and breast cancer, *Cancer,* 33, 174, 1974.

80. **Masters, J. R. W., Hawkins, R. A., Sangster, K. et al.,** Oestrogen receptors, cellularity, elastosis and menstrual status in human breast cancer, *Eur. J. Cancer,* 14, 303, 1978.

81. **Fisher, E. R., Redmond, C. K., Liu, H., et al.,** Correlation of estrogen receptor and pathological characteristics of invasive breast cancer, *Cancer,* 45, 349, 1980.

82. **Masters, J. R. W., Millis, R. R., King, R. J. B., et al.,** Elastosis and response to endocrine therapy in human breast cancer, *Br. J. Cancer,* 39, 536, 1979.

83. **Reyes, M. G., Bazile, D. B., Tosch, T., and Rubenstone, A. I.,** Periductal elastic tissue of breast cancer: quantitative histologic study, *Arch. Pathol. Lab. Med.,* 106, 610, 1982.

84. **Underwood, J. C. E.,** Lymphoreticular infiltration in human tumours: prognostic and biological implications: a review, *Br. J. Cancer,* 30, 538, 1974.

85. **Silva, J. S., Cox, C. E., Wells, S. A. et al.,** Biochemical correlates of morphologic differentiation in human breast cancer, *Surgery,* 92, 443, 1982.

86. **Ghosh, L., Ghosh, B. C., and Dasgupta, T. K.,** Immunocytological localisation of estrogen in human mammary carcinoma cells by horseradish-anti-horseradish peroxidase complex, *J. Surg. Oncol.,* 10, 221, 1978.

87. **Lee, S. H.,** Cytochemical study of estrogen receptor in human mammary cancer, *Am. J. Clin. Pathol.,* 70, 197, 1978.

88. **Pertschuk, L. P., Tobin, E. H., Brigati, D. J., et al.,** Immunofluorescent detection of estrogen receptors in breast cancer, *Cancer,* 41, 907, 1978.

89. **Pertschuk, L. P., Gaetjens, E., Carter, A. C. et al.,** An improved histochemical assay for detection of estrogen receptor in mammary cancer: comparison with biochemical assay, *Am. J. Clin. Pathol.,* 71, 504, 1979.

90. **Berger, G., Frappart, L., Berger, N. et al.,** Localisation cytoplasmique des recepteurs steroidiens des carcinomes mammaires par histofluorescence, *Arch. Anat. Cytol. Pathol.,* 28, 341, 1980.

91. **Mercer, W. D., Lippman, M. E., Wahl, T. M. et al.,** The use of immunocytochemical techniques for the detection of steroid hormones in breast cancer cells, *Cancer,* 46, 2859, 1980.

92. **Rao, B. R., Fry, C. G., Hunt, S. et al.,** A fluorescent probe for rapid detection of estrogen receptors, *Cancer,* 46, 2902, 1980.

93. **Eusebi, V., Cerasoli, P. T., Guidelli-Guidi, S. et al.,** A two-stage immunocytochemical method for estrogen receptor analysis: correlation with morphologic parameters of breast carcinomas, *Tumori,* 56, 315, 1981.

94. **Tominaga, T., Kitamura, M., Saito, T. et al.,** Comparative histochemical and biochemical assays of estrogen receptors in breast cancer patients, *Gann,* 72, 60, 1981.

95. **Hanna, W., Ryder, D. E., and Mobbs, B. G.,** Cellular localisation of estrogen binding sites in human breast cancer, *Am. J. Clin. Pathol.,* 77, 391, 1982.

96. **Lee, S. H.,** The histochemistry of estrogen receptors, *Histochemistry,* 71, 491, 1981.

97. **Raam, S., Nemeth, E., Tamura, H. et al.,** Immunohistochemical localisation of estrogen receptors in human mammary carcinoma using antibodies to the receptor proteins, *Eur. J. Cancer Clin. Oncol.,* 18, 1, 1982.

98. **Penney, G. C. and Hawkins, R. A.,** Histochemical detection of estrogen receptors: a progress report, *Br. J. Cancer,* 45, 237, 1982.

99. **Underwood, J. C. E., Sher, E., Reed, M. et al.,** Biochemical assessment of histochemical methods for oestrogen receptor localisation, *J. Clin. Pathol.,* 35, 401, 1982.

100. **Kurzon, R. M. and Sternberger, L. A.,** Estrogen receptor immunocytochemistry, *J. Histochem. Cytochem.,* 26, 803, 1978.

101. **Nenci, I., Beccati, M. D., Piffanelli, A., and Lanza, G.,** Detection and dynamic localization of estradiol-receptor complexes in intact target cells by immunoflourescence technique, *J. Steroid Biochem.,* 7, 505, 1976.

102. **Nenci, I., Dandliker, W. B., Meyers, C. Y. et al.,** Estrogen receptor cytochemistry by fluorescent estrogen, *J. Histochem. Cytochem.,* 28, 1081, 1980.
103. **Pertschuk, L. P., Tobin, E. H., Gaetjens, E. et al.,** Histochemical assay of estrogen and progesterone receptor in breast cancer: correlation with biochemical assays and patient response to endocrine therapies, *Cancer,* 46, 2896, 1980.
104. **Pertschuk, L. P., Gaetjens, E., Carter, A. C. et al.,** Histochemistry of steroid receptors in breast cancer, *Ann. Clin. Lab. Sci.,* 9, 219, 1979.
105. **Pertschuk, L. P.,** Detection of estrogen binding in human mammary carcinoma by immunofluorescence: a new technique utilizing the binding hormone in a polymerized state, *Res. Comm. Chem. Pathol. Pharmacol.,* 17, 771, 1976.
106. **Walker, R. A., Cove, D. H., and Howell, A.,** Histological detection of estrogen receptors in human breast carcinomas, *Lancet,* 1, 171, 1980.
107. **Taylor, C. R., Cooper, C. L., Kurman, R. J. et al.,** Detection of estrogen receptor in breast and endometrial carcinoma by the immunoperoxidase technique, *Cancer,* 47, 2634, 1981.
108. **Morrow, B., Leav, I., Delellis, R. A., and Raam, S.,** Use of polyestradiol phosphate and anti-17β estradiol antibodies for the localization of estrogen receptor in target tissues: a critique, *Cancer,* 46, 2872, 1980.
109. **Fishman, J. and Fishman, J. H.,** Competitive binding assay for estradiol receptor using immobilized antibody, *J. Clin. Endocrinol. Metab.,* 39, 603, 1974.
110. **Casteneda, E. and Liao, S.,** The use of anti-steroid antibodies in the characterization of steroid receptors, *J. Biol. Chem.,* 250, 883, 1975.
111. **McCarty, K. S., Jr., Reintgen, D. S., Seigler, H. F., and McCarty, K. S., Sr.,** Cytochemistry of sex steroid receptors: a critique, *Br. Cancer Res. Treat.,* 1, 315, 1982.
112. **Zehr, D. R., Sataswaroop, P. G., and Sheehan, D. M.,** Nonspecific staining in the immunolocalisation of oestrogen receptors, *J. Steroid Biochem.,* 14, 613, 1981.
113. **Mercer, W. D., Edwards, D. P., Chamness, G. C., and McGuire, W. L.,** Failure of estradiol immunofluorescence in MCF-7 breast cancer cells to detect estrogen receptors, *Cancer Res.,* 41, 4644, 1981.
114. **Mercer, W. D., Carlsen, C. A., Wahl, T. M., and Teague, P. O.,** Identification of estrogen receptor in mammary carcinoma cells by immunofluorescence, *Am. J. Clin. Pathol.,* 70, 330, 1978.
115. **McCarty, K. S., Jr., Woodard, B. H., Nichols, D. E. et al.,** Comparison of biochemical and histochemical techniques for estrogen receptor analysis in mammary carcinoma, *Cancer,* 46, 2842, 1980.
116. **Dandliker, W. B., Levison, S. A., and Brown, R. J.,** Hormone binding by cells and cell fragments as visualized by fluorescence microscopy, *Res. Comm. Chem. Pathol. Pharmacol.,* 14, 103, 1976.
117. **Dandliker, W. B., Hicks, A. N., Levison, S. A., and Brawn, R. J.,** A fluorescein-labelled derivative of oestradiol with binding affinity towards cellular receptors, *Biochem. Biophys. Res. Comm.,* 74, 538, 1977.
118. **Barrows, G. H., Stroupe, S. B., and Riehm, J. D.,** Nuclear uptake of ethyl-succinamide bridged 17β estradiol-fluorescein as a marker of estrogen activity, *Am. J. Clin. Pathol.,* 73, 330, 1980.
119. **Dandliker, W. B., Brawn, R. J., Hsu, M.-L. et al.,** Investigations of hormone-receptor interactions by means of fluorescence labelling, *Cancer Res.,* 38, 4212, 1978.

# INDEX

## A

Acetone fixation, 138
Adenocarcinomas, 47
Albumin chase, 5
Albumin-estradiol conjugates, 158
Albumin washes, 9
Androgen receptors, 94, 106—108
  DCC assays of, see Dextran-coated charcoal
    assays
  DCC vs. fluorescent assessments of, 95, 97
  determining positivity of, 95, 98
  factors affecting detection of, 95, 97—98
  fluorescent conjugate determination of, see Flu-
    orescent conjugate techniques
  heterogeneity of, 106—107
  histochemical techniques for, see Histochemical
    techniques
  nuclear binding and, 98
  as predictor of clinical response, 94, 98, 103
  problems in detection of, 94, 107
  prostatic acid phosphatase and, 107—108
  specificity and, 95
Autoradiography, see Radioautography

## B

Benign prostatic hyperplasia (BPH), see also Pros-
    tate cancers, 106
Binding capacity, see Competition experiments;
    Saturability
Binding ligands, see Ligands; specific ligands
Biochemical techniques, see also specific techniques
  in combination with histochemical techniques,
    28—30, 108
  correlation of with clinical response, 154
  correlation of with fluorescent techniques, 40, 42,
    86—88, 143—144
  in demonstration of type I binding, 86, 119—120
  correlation of with histochemical technique, 40,
    88—90, 124—129
  determining positivity with, see Positivity,
    determining
    factors affecting, 17, 20
  fluorescent techniques vs., 114—115
  heterogeneous results with, 65
  histochemical techniques vs., 156
    for androgen receptors, 94
    for estrogen receptors, 16, 17, 20, 38, 42—43,
      79, 88—90, 115
    for prostate cancers, 105—106, 108
    size of tissue required, 68, 70, 80
  procedures for, 151—152
  radioautography vs., 7, 9
  sequential assessments with, 76
  tumor cellularity and, 155
Bovine serum albumin (BSA), see also Fluorescent
    conjugate techniques, 39

## C

Breast cancer, see Mammary tumors

Cancers, see specific cancers
Capacity, see Competition experiments; Saturability
Chemotherapy, clinical response to, 154
  hormone responsiveness as predictor of, 56—59,
    76—79, 124, 154
  factors affecting, 58
Clinical response, see specific therapies and
    treatments
Competition experiments, see also Saturability,
    Specificity
  in fluorescent conjugate studies, 119—120, 158
    6-FE vs. 17-FE, 31
  with fluorescent peroxidase techniques, 138, 140,
    143
  inhibitor concentration and, 157
Coumestrol, 158
Cytochemical techniques, see also specific tech-
    niques, 45—46

## D

Dextran-coated charcoal (DCC) assays
  accuracy of, 38
  advantages and disadvantages of, 124
  correlation of with fluorescent conjugate
    techniques
    for androgen receptors, 95, 97
    on determining ER status, 125, 126
    discrepancies between, 126—129
  correlation of with fluorescent peroxidase tech-
    niques, 143—144
  correlation of with immunoperoxidase techniques,
    135
  determining positivity with, see Positivity,
    determining
  ERICA techniques vs., 21, 24
  fluorescent conjugate techniques vs., 17
  problems with, 153
  procedures for, 122, 151—152
  saturability and, 151—152
  sensitivity, 25, 27—30
  specificity, 25, 27—30
  usefulness of, 153
Diethylstilbestrol (DES), see Endocrine therapy

## E

Elastosis, 155
  grading of, 122
Encroachment phenomenon, 46, 47
Endocrine therapy

chemotherapy vs., 124
factors affecting clinical response to, 38, 52, 58
predicting clinical response to
  biochemical vs. histochemical techniques for,
    129
  combined techniques for, 25—30, 88
  DCC assays for, 25, 27—28
  ERICA for, 25
  fluorescent conjugate techniques for, 25, 27,
    30
  hormone responsiveness in, 56—59, 75—80,
    86, 88—90, 124, 150
  nuclear-bound 17-FE for, 33
  progesterone receptors for, 28—29
  radioautography for, 7, 10—11
predicting clinical response to in post-mastectomy
  tumors
  hormone responsiveness in, 76—79
predicting clinical response to in prostate cancers
  androgen receptors in, 94, 98, 103, 104, 108
  combined measures for, 108
  estrogen receptors in, 103—104
  heterogeneity as tool in, 106
  histochemical studies for, 104
  types of in Chinese study, 53
Endometrial carcinomas, 47
ERICA, see Estrogen receptor immunocytochemical
  assay
ER status, see also Hormone responsiveness
  correlation of
    with age, 122
    with clinical response, 154
    with menstrual status, 153—154
    with tumor characteristics, 121—122, 154—
     155
  determining positivity of, see Positivity,
    determining
  importance of in treatment of mammary tumors,
    88
  prediction of
    mean nuclear areas, in, 155
    with morphometric features, 122—124
  as predictor of clinical response, see specific ther-
    apies and treatments
17β-Estradiol-6-carboxymethyl oxime-BSA FITC,
  see Fluorescent conjugate techniques
16β-Estradiol-17-hemisuccinyl-bovine serum albumin-fluorescein isothiocyanate (17-FE), see
  Fluorescent conjugate techniques
Estrogen binding, see also Estrogen receptors
  histological differentiation and, 143
  mechanism of, 152
Estrogen receptor immunocytochemical assay
  (ERICA)
  DCC techniques vs., 21, 24
  detection of type I estrogen receptors and, 24—25
  for estrogen receptors, 104
  fluorescent conjugate techniques vs., 21, 105
  nuclear localization and, 21
  procedures for, 21
  sensitivity, 25

specificity, 24, 25
Estrogen receptors, see also ER status; Estrogen
  binding
  activation of, 152
  association of with progesterone receptors, 43,
    45, 53
  biochemical vs. histochemical localization of, 79,
    115
  biochemical measurement of, see Biochemical
    techniques
  detection of type I, 16, 24—25
  DCC measurement of, see Dextran-coated char-
    coal assays
  determining positivity of, 38, 43, 66—67, 89—
    90, 104, 125
    with fluorescent conjugate techniques, see Flu-
     orescent conjugate techniques; Fluorescent
     peroxidase conjugate techniques
  heterogeneity of in mammary tumors, 7, 150
  histochemical techniques for, see Histochemical
    techniques
  in mouse uterus, 4
  multiple sites for, 26—27, 90, 114, 115, 119,
    152
    biochemical vs. fluorescent definition of,
     114—115, 125
    as diagnostic tool, 33
    evidence for, 20, 105
    6-FE vs. 17-FE, 31
    in prostate cancers, 104—105
  nuclear vs. cytoplasm as location of, 21, 23
  in prostate cancers, see Prostate cancers
  radioautography of, see Radioautography
Ethanol/acetone fixation, 138

## F

6-FE, see Fluorescent conjugate techniques
17-FE, see Fluorescent conjugate techniques
Fluorescent conjugate techniques
  advantages and disadvantages of, 80, 134, 158
  for androgen receptors
    clinical response and, see specific therapies and
     treatments; specific tumors
    factors affecting detection of, 95, 97—98, 107
    specificity, 95
  biochemical techniques vs., 114—115
  competitive binding and, see Competition
    experiments
  correlation of with biochemical techniques, 40,
    42, 86—88
    in demonstration of type I binding, 86, 119—
     120
  correlation of with DCC assays, 17
    for androgen receptors, 95, 97
    on determining ER status, 125, 126
    discrepancies between, 126—129
  correlation of with response to endocrine therapy,
    86, 88—90
  DCC assays vs., 17

demonstration of type II binding in, 120—121
description of fluorescing cells and, 114
determining positivity with, see Positivity,
    determining
effects of incubation times, 119—120
ERICA techniques vs., 21, 105
fluorescence variation and, 116—117
heterogeneity of results with, 64—66
interpretation of, 45
ligands for
    concentration of, 31, 42, 114, 115, 118—119,
        157, 158
    coupling sites and, 135
    6-FE vs. 17-FE, 16—17, 30—32, 104—105,
        135—136
    relative binding of, 17, 159
in malignant effusions, 45—46
peroxidase conjugation vs., 137
procedures for
    with androgen receptors, 94
    in Canadian studies, 86—87
    in Chinese studies, 52—53
    criticisms of, 38, 42—43
    effects of freezing and storage on, 115—116
    in Italian studies, 64, 66—67
reagent stability and, 151
reproducibility of, 79
sensitivity, 25, 27—30
specificity, 25, 27—30, 46, 116—121
typical findings with, 39
usefulness of, 38, 47, 48, 59
validation of, 40, 42
Fluorescent peroxidase conjugate techniques
    advantages and disadvantages of, 144
    binding efficiency, 136
    correlation of with biochemical techniques, 143—
        144
    correlation of with tumor characteristics, 143
    distribution of staining in, 139—143
    fluorescein conjugation in vs., 137
    ligands for
        concentrations of, 138—139
        preparation of, 136—137
    procedures for
        staining methods for, 138—139
        tissue preparation for, 137—138

## G

Glutaraldehyde method, 136—137, 144
Gross cystic disease fluid protein (GCDFP-15), 155

## H

Histochemical techniques, see also specific
        techniques
    advantages and disadvantages of, 16—17, 124—
        125, 134

antibody method, see also Immunofluorescence
        assay; Immunohistochemical techniques
    advantages and disadvantages of, 157—159
    biochemical techniques vs., 156
        for androgen receptors, 94
        for estrogen receptors, 16, 17, 20, 38, 42—43,
            79, 88—90, 115
        for prostate cancers, 105—106, 108
        size of tissue required, 68, 70, 80
    clinical response and, see specific therapies and
        treatments
    combined with biochemical techniques, 28—30
    correlation of with biochemical techniques, 40,
        88—90, 124—129
        factors affecting, 17, 20
    with cytologic material, 79
    determining positivity with, see Positivity,
        determining
    interpretation of, 48
    labeled ligand method, see also Fluorescent con-
        jugate techniques; Fluorescent conjugate per-
        oxidase technique, 158
    procedures for, 47, 48
    sucrose density gradient analyses vs., 157, 158
    usefulness of, 47
    validation of, 151, 156
Hormone responsiveness, see also ER status
    biology of in mammary tumors, 46—47
    clinical utility of, 150
    correlation of
        with age, 54, 55, 59, 67, 69, 80
        with disease progress, 80
        with disease stage, 54, 59
        with lymph node involvement, 68, 71
        with menstruation status, 54, 55, 58—59, 67,
            68
        with tumor characteristics, 54—55, 59, 67, 68,
            70—78
        with tumor size during perimenopausal period,
            80
    of cytologic material, 79
    determining positivity of, see Positivity,
        determining
    factors affecting, 58, 153
    in paramenopausal women, 154
    as predictor of clinical response, see specific ther-
        apies and treatments
    variability of in primary vs. secondary lesions,
        56, 58
Hormone therapies, see also Endocrine therapy
    clinical response to, 154
    in prostate cancers, 94
Horseradish peroxidase
    advantages and disadvantages of, 134—135
    as conjugate, see also Fluorescent conjugate tech-
        niques, 136
11β-Hydroxyprogesterone hemisuccinate-BSA tetra-
        methylrhodamine isothiocyanate, see Flu-
        orescent conjugate techniques

## I

Immunocytochemical techniques, see also Estrogen
    receptor immunocytochemical assay, 157—
    158
Immunofluorescence assay, 107—108
Immunohistochemical techniques, 65—66
Immunoperoxidase techniques
    correlation of with DCC assays, 135
    problems with, 135
    procedures for, 134—135
    specificity, 135

## L

Leiomyosarcoma of prostate, 106
Ligands
    concentration of, 31, 42, 114, 115, 118—119,
        138—139, 157, 158
    coupling sites and, 135
    6-FE vs. 17-FE, 16—17, 30—32, 104—105,
        135—136
    preparation of, 136—137
    relative binding of, 17, 159

## M

Malignant effusions, 45—46
Mammary tumors
    clinical response in, see also specific therapies
        and treatments
        combined measures as predictor of, 25—30, 88
        criteria for, 53
        DCC assays as predictor of, 25, 27—28
        ERICA as predictor of, 25
        fluorescent techniques as predictor of, 25, 27,
          30
        nuclear 17-FE as predictor of, 33
        progesterone receptors as predictor of, 28—29
    defining positivity in, see Positivity, determining
    estrogen receptors in, see Estrogen receptors
    heterogeneity in, 116—117
    hormone responsiveness in, see also Hormone
        responsiveness
        biology of, 46—47
    morphometric classification of, 122—124
    nuclear 17-FE as indicator of survival in, 33
    in paramenopausal women, 153—154
Mean nuclear area calculation, 122—124
    usefulness of, 155
Monoclonal antibodies, see also Estrogen receptor
    immunocytochemical assay, 158—159
Morphometric classification, 122—124

## N

Needle aspiration, usefulness of, 64

Nuclear acceptor, 152
Nuclear translocation, see Translocation

## O

O-BSA-FITC, see Fluorescent conjugate techniques
Ovarian cancers, 47

## P

PBS washes, 16, 21
Periodate method, 136—137, 144
Peroxidase conjugation, see also Fluorescent peroxi-
    dase conjugate techniques, 144
Phosphate buffered saline (PBS) wash, 16, 21
Pleural effusions, 45—46
Positivity, determining, 52, 53, 57—58, 66—67
    for androgen receptors, 95, 98
    for estrogen receptors, 38, 43, 66—67, 89—90,
        104, 125
Post-staining washes, see also specific washes, 42
Progesterone-binding protein (PBP), 155—156
Progesterone receptors, 155—156
    association of with estrogen receptors, 43, 45, 53
    correlation of with tumor characteristics, 154
    in prediction of clinical response, 28—29
Prostate cancers
    androgen receptors in, 94, 106—107
        correlation of PAP with, 107—108
        DCC vs. fluorescent assessments of, 95, 97
        determining positivity of, see Positivity,
          determining
        factors affecting detection of, 95, 97—98
        heterogeneity of binding of, 106—107
        problems measuring, 94
        specificity, 95
    clinical response in, see specific therapies and
        treatments
    estrogen receptors in, 47, 103—104
        determining positivity of, see Positivity,
          determining
        multiple sites for, 104—105
    heterogeneity of steroid bindings in, 106
Prostate carcinosarcomas, 106
Prostatic acid phosphatase (PAP) and androgen
    binding, 107

## R

Radioautography, 2—11
    advantages and disadvantages of, 2
    biochemical techniques vs., 7, 9
    detection of low ER levels with, 9
    determining positivity with, see Positivity,
        determining
    for estrogen binding studies, 4—5
    for malignant tumors, 6—9
    for nuclear type II sites, 9

procedures for
chemicals in, 2
identification of target cells, 3
thaw-mount techniques, 2—3
tissues used in, 2—3
specificity, 5
usefulness of
for localization of sites, 10
for predicting clinical response, 11
Receptors, see specific receptors
Regression, definition of, 43
Responsiveness, see Hormone responsiveness
$R_f$, see Hormone responsiveness

## S

Saturability, see also Competition experiments; specific techniques, 157
demonstrating by type of receptors, 152—153
Sensitivity, see also specific techniques, 151
Specificity, see also Competition experiments; specific techniques, 151
demonstrating by type of receptors, 152—153
Steroid receptors, see specific receptors
Stromal invasion, 155
Sucrose density gradient (SDG) techniques, 38, 152
determining positivity with, see Positivity, determining

histochemical techniques vs., 157, 158
problems with, 153
usefulness of, 153

## T

Thaw-mount autoradiography, see Radioautography
Translocation, 152
cytoplasmic type II estrogen receptors and, 31
demonstration of, 24
detection of with fluorescent peroxidase techniques, 140
heat induction of, 31—32, 98
with immunocytochemical methods, 157
process of, 21
in type III sites, 153
Tumors, see Mammary tumors; Prostate cancers; specific cancers

## W

Washes, see specific washes

## X

X-ray therapy, clinical response to, 75—79